Connections in the Clinic

Randall Reitz · Laura E. Sudano ·
Mark P. Knudson
Editors

Connections in the Clinic

Relational Narratives from Team-Based
Primary Care

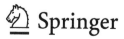 Springer

Editors
Randall Reitz
St. Mary's Family Medicine Residency
Grand Junction, CO, USA

Laura E. Sudano
Department of Family Medicine
University of California
San Diego, CA, USA

Mark P. Knudson
Department of Family and Community
Medicine
Wake Forest University
Winston-Salem, NC, USA

ISBN 978-3-030-46276-5   ISBN 978-3-030-46274-1   (eBook)
https://doi.org/10.1007/978-3-030-46274-1

This Springer imprint is published by the registered company Springer Nature Switzerland AG
The registered company address is: Gewerbestrasse 11, 6330 Cham, Switzerland

Randall to Ana
We run through life
Round the same lakes
I push the gas
You pump the brakes

Laura
For those before and after me.

Mark to Jenni
who has shared a life, taught me about life,
helped me weather the hardships and
appreciate the joys of life, and blessed me in
supporting the lives of 3 amazing children.

Preface

I'm often drawn to write haiku about the constellation Orion. I usually phrase these thoughts as anthropomorphic salutations to the heavens:

Body, limbs, belt, bow
May your lasting grit and grace
Guide my path today

I've reflected on why I do this with Orion, but never with other equally beautiful patterns in the stars. I've arrived at 2 conclusions: First, I prefer Orion because I have imbued within him many of the values and strengths that I desire for myself. But, perhaps more importantly and more basically, I identify with Orion because I can identify Orion. Of the billions of stars visible in the night sky, the pattern that we call Orion is one of the few that I have internalized. I trust that during the winter months, he will always be overhead in the early morning.

Gentle Orion
Float above the wood stack
Light my home this dawn

This doesn't mean that other stars or patterns are less visible or less striking. It simply means that I don't recognize them as patterns. While others see dragons, scorpions, dogs, and bears in the sky, I've only made sense of the seven or so stars that we call Orion. I have come to connect these dots in a way that renders them memorable and meaningful to me. I have created and recreated a personal narrative around these inanimate objects.

Orion hovers south
Then fades in the blaze of the
Grand Mesa sunrise

This is the power of narrative. Our daily life is so full of events and observations that we are unable to assimilate all of it. As a result, we create shortcuts to help us make sense of the deluge of data. Over time, these connections take on a meaning of their own and result in a story that explains the importance of what was previously a random assortment of events.

Perhaps more importantly, if we fail to create connections between the stimuli of our 5 senses, then in a very real way, the stimuli never happens. Events that aren't connected into narratives are easily overlooked as random occurrences. But, when we encircle them within a story, we find meaning in them and wisdom for how to approach a similar constellation of information in the future.

Connections in the Clinic is an attempt to find meaning in the relationships that are created in team-based primary care. These stories and images aim to help us make sense of the more poignant experiences in the clinical context and of the events outside the clinic that shape our approach to health care. Without collecting these narratives into one volume, we would each only have one or two constellations to make sense of our experiences. But, by collecting and organizing them, we begin to recognize and appreciate the full diversity of the patterns across our lives.

I hope that reading these stories will inspire your work and relationships.

Grand Junction, USA   Randall Reitz

* * *

This book is as broad and grand as the constellations above us, encompassing the expanse of the human condition from birth to death. Yet it is also as specific as the relationship between 2 people, which we experience in caring for others. We hope readers find meaning in this scope of stories, and in the emotional reflection that is captured in each of the narratives and poems.

As the first submissions for this book were coming in, I experienced the death of a dear 91-year-old patient I had cared for over 20 years. Her last weeks of hospice care were full of daily interactions with her and her daughter from England. The sadness of loss was profound, as our "doctor–patient" relationship was complex and atypical. From the start, my quiet professionalism was greeted with her argumentative combative style. She challenged every medication I proposed, questioned every diagnosis I considered. But I slowly learned that she valued my role, and would take the medications or follow up for the tests she had argued against.

In her last weeks, she softened greatly, reflecting on the medical care we had shared. One day, she looked at me and said, "For years you have heard my complaints, listened as I bragged about my daughter, sat quietly as I railed about politics, and looked with interest on the pictures I shared of my 2 grandchildren.

Now that I am almost gone, it's time for you to tell me about you!" We spent the next half hour, talking, and she attended to every word of my story about my family, my struggles, and my joys. She teared up when I told her of my child's battle with death the previous year, interjecting, "I remember last year, you seemed both distant and more compassionate than I ever remembered. I feel selfish for not realizing that when I had pain, I was not always alone."

Yet in her last days, she kept her sense of humor (sarcastic, ironic, and sincere). In an email she sent a picture of her hospice dinner: pureed asparagus and lime sherbet. "They won't have to wait until death for my body to turn moldy green!" She also retained her authoritative style, telling me that I should spend more time writing. We had shared a love of poetry by Philip Levine who died that February. She sent me the New Yorker, dedicated to him, with admonition that he gave up a good career in Detroit to become a poet. "If Medicine doesn't work out, maybe you could go to Iowa, and learn to write. I am certain that I have given you a few decades of stuff to write about!"

Months after her funeral, I found myself at a local cemetery one winter eve, and realized she was buried there. I teared up at the thought of her death. I struggled with the larger issues of loss. And then, I was reminded of her energy, her enthusiasm, her sarcastic and pervasive sense of humor, and I realized that she was not turning green in a pine box buried there. Her spirit lived on, to enliven those who remember her.

Untitled

Frozen fiddle strings of icy air, high pitched
and tendril thin, found their way
thru button hole, up cuffs
and down collar past heavy scarf.

Standing on the hillock of dead grass,
black sky with paucity of stars
was no longer a blanket of darkness,
but instead an empty door to the cold and vastness
of the universe.

I looked back,
across thousands of granite markers
and imagined the fresh earth that covered
pine boards,
remembered the last shovel of dirt
and the hollow sound it made,
imagined the loneliness and emptiness
of a thousand boxes,
and knew that you were in none of them.

We hope that our readers find a pause at these stories and poems that explore our interactions with those we heal, our relationships with mentors and family who teach and guide us in our healing art, and our introspections into who we are as healers. We trust that many of you will make it a regular habit to explore the narratives and poetry of other healers, and that some number of you might be inspired to use writing as a powerful reflective tool of your own.

Winston-Salem, USA   Mark P. Knudson

* * *

What just happened? I thought, after hanging up the phone with my mom. "He left you to die," and described, "When you opened the door, you looked like death." There was a coordination of care, an understanding that my husband needed to return to work after being with me for those few weeks in the hospital being treated for what was thought to be viral meningitis. It turned out that I had contracted a bacteria that destroyed my heart valve and distributed emboli on my vital organs, including my brain.

She just shared her account of my near-death experience. Her re-telling of the story, however, was not my story. In fact, it wasn't my experience at all. Her truth was not my truth, but it was her truth nonetheless.

But what was my story? How could I articulate what happened to me during the course of my illness? The medical complications, the medical team's care, and the family conflict? Better yet, how could I make sense out of this nonsense life event, and how did it change me—my approach to patient care, education, and relationships?

This is what narrative medicine means to me. That I can integrate an experience I had into my identity as a person, a professional, through the use of storytelling. This mixing allows for one to reflect and describe the experience. The reader is exposed to the story, and sometimes the wisdom and knowledge that the events inspired in you become exposed in a way that the reader may share your wisdom and knowledge.

After my medical experience, I considered how we can invite others to share experiences such as these and how we can use them as educational tools. I approached, or more like cornered, Randall after a plenary session during an annual conference and asked him if he would be interested in developing this idea. The training of healthcare providers, the awareness of treating the whole family, and the healthcare landscape has changed since the edited book, The Shared Experience of Illness (McDaniel, Hepworth, & Doberty, 1997). But how far have we come in implementing best practices and affecting change?

Storytelling is unique in that we, as humans, can express it through art or language. Some say that storytelling is as old as time. One of the first accounts of storytelling can be traced back to somewhere between 15000 and 13000 BC. Children in the Pyrenees Mountains found drawings of over 2000 figures with elements of a narrative (Lockett, 2007). Homer's epics are a popular example of storytelling, which were originally told by Homer around 1200 BC and were written about 700 BC.

People tell stories and listen to them because there is conflict and some sort of resolution, albeit painful at times. And through that, they see the knowledge gained and sometimes that knowledge resonates with them, and they carry that knowledge home. Told right, storytelling doesn't tell you the lesson learned. It shows you.

These narratives shared in this book, along with its images, will hopefully inspire you to integrate your experiences and create your story so that one day you may share your truth with someone.

San Diego, USA   Laura E. Sudano

Acknowledgments

This book shares stories of relationships—some good, some bad. We're fortunate to have benefited from many good relationships—many of which are similar to those described in the chapters of this book.

Teachers and Mentors have guided our professional development, helped us to avoid mishaps, and helped us to clean up when we didn't avoid them. Randall wishes to acknowledge Wendy Watson, Steve Hurd, Larry Mauksch, Colleen Fogarty, Jeff Ring, and Deb Taylor. Laura wishes to acknowledge Randall Reitz, Mark P. Knudson, Richard Lord, and Jo Ellen Patterson for their steadfast support. Mark wishes to acknowledge Robin Blake who first introduced him to literature and medicine, and Paul Gross and everyone at Pulse, who have nurtured the love of narrative medicine.

Family is our first social foyer in which we learn connection with others. We are grateful to our families of origin and families of creation without whom we could not be self-reflective and grow.

Patients are what drew us to our occupations, as we dreamed of helping others. But somewhere along the path of providing care, we realized that patients were our ultimate teacher, baring their souls to us to give us an understanding of the human condition, and helping us to realize the important healing power of the shared, spoken, and written word.

Colleagues and Collaborators have blessed us across our careers and helped to make this book possible. We'd like to send our appreciation to the authors and illustrators who undertook this process with us. Your lives, stories, and your ability to write stories about your lives inspire us. We are all medical educators and have been blessed with excellent faculty colleagues and trainees. You have enriched our days and helped us to contribute to the scholarship and workforce of our fields.

And finally, we want to express our gratitude for the great support from the staff of Springer Publishers.

Contents

Editors and Contributors

About the Editors

Randall Reitz, PhD, LMFT is the Director of Behavioral Medicine at the St. Mary's Family Medicine Residency in Grand Junction, Colorado. He completed his doctoral studies at Brigham Young University. Outside of work, he serves on the Grand Junction City Council, enjoys trail running with his wife, mountain biking with his children, and baking with his thoughts.

Laura E. Sudano, PhD, LMFT is the Associate Director for Integrated Behavioral Health and behavioral science faculty at the University of California, San Diego. She completed a doctorate in Human Development with emphasis in Marriage and Family Therapy at Virginia Polytechnic Institute and State University (Virginia Tech) in 2015. Outside of work, she enjoys being active with her family and friends.

Mark P. Knudson, MD is the Vice Chair in the Department of Family and Community Medicine of Wake Forest University School of Medicine, in Winston-Salem, North Carolina. He completed his medical degree at the University of Virginia, and his Family Medicine Residency and Fellowship at University of Missouri-Columbia. Outside of work, he enjoys biking, hiking, and spending time with his wife and 3 children.

Contributors

Claudia W. Allen Department of Family Medicine, University of Virginia, Charlottesville, VA, USA

Jennifer L. Ayres Still River Counseling, PLLC, Austin, TX, USA

Jamie E. Banker California Lutheran University, Thousand Oaks, CA, USA

Lisa Black Department of Family Medicine, University of California San Diego Family Medicine, San Diego, CA, USA

David C. Conway NH Dartmouth Family Medicine Residency (Retired), Concord, NH, USA

Amy L. Davis Colorado Mesa University, Grand Junction, CO, USA

Keith S. Dickerson St. Mary's Family Medicine Residency, Grand Junction, CO, USA

Deborah Edberg Department of Family Medicine, Rush University, Chicago, IL, USA

Colleen T. Fogarty Department of Family Medicine, University of Rochester, Rochester, NY, USA

Kathryn Fraser Halifax Health Family Medicine Residency Program, Daytona Beach, FL, USA

Cameron Froude Bliss in Being Family Therapy, San Francisco, CA, USA

Sarah G. Gerrish Family Medicine Residency of Idaho, Boise, ID, USA

Arnold Goldberg Brown Family Medicine, West Warwick, RI, USA

Lucy Graham St. Mary's Family Medicine Residency, Grand Junction, CO, USA

Kathryn W. Hart Marillac Health, Grand Junction, CO, USA

Jennifer Hodgson Medical Family Therapy Doctoral Program, East Carolina University, Greenville, NC, USA

Rachel L. Hughes Antioch University - Seattle, Auburn, WA, USA

Laurie C. Ivey University of Denver Graduate School of Professional Psychology, Denver, CO, USA

Ajantha Jayabarathan Coral Shared-Care Health Center, Halifax, NS, Canada

Michelle K. Keating Wake Forest School of Medicine, Winstom-Salem, NC, USA

Mark P. Knudson Wake Forest School of Medicine, Winston-Salem, NC, USA

Angela L. Lamson East Carolina University, Greenville, NC, USA

Juli Larsen Grand Junction, CO, USA

Florencia Lebensohn-Chialvo University of San Diego, San Diego, CA, USA

Alan Lorenz University of Rochester, Rochester, NY, USA

Alice Yuxi Lu University of Massachusetts Medical School, Worcester, MA, USA

Julie Lynn Mayer Swarthmore, PA, USA

Larry B. Mauksch Department of Family Medicine (Emeritus), University of Washington, Seattle, WA, USA

Justin H. McCarthy St. Mary's Family Medicine Residency, Grand Junction, CO, USA

Tai J. Mendenhall University of Minnesota, Minneapolis/Saint Paul, MN, USA

Sabrina Mitchell St. Mary's Family Medicine Residency, Grand Junction, CO, USA

Stephen W.B. Mitchell Create Your Couple Story, Denver, CO, USA

Samantha Pelican Monson Denver Health Medical Center, Denver, CO, USA

Glenda Mutinda JPS Health Network, Ft. Worth, TX, USA

Amy J. Odom Sparrow/Michigan State University Family Medicine Residency, Lansing, MI, USA

Michael Olson St. Mary's Family Medicine Residency, Grand Junction, CO, USA

Cormac A. O'Donovan Wake Forest School of Medicine, Winston-Salem, NC, USA

Randall Reitz St. Mary's Family Medicine Residency, Grand Junction, CO, USA

Jeffrey Ring Glendale, CA, USA

Tania Riosvelasco Hamburg, Germany

Amy M. Romain Sparrow/Michigan State University Family Medicine Residency, Lansing, MI, USA

Christine Runyan Department of Family Medicine, University of Massachusetts Medical School, Worcester, MA, USA

Julia Sager Maine Medical Center Preventive Medicine Residency, Portland, ME, USA

John Scheid Denver, CO, USA

Alexandra Schmidt Hulst Rocky Mountain Health Plans, Grand Junction, CO, USA

David B. Seaburn University of Rochester Medical Center, Rochester, NY, USA

Karlynn Sievers St. Mary's Family Medicine Residency, Grand Junction, CO, USA

Paul D. Simmons St. Mary's Family Medicine Residency, Grand Junction, CO, USA

John G. Spangler Wake Forest School of Medicine, Winston-Salem, NC, USA

Sally Stratford Grand Junction, CO, USA

Laura E. Sudano Department of Family Medicine, University of California San Diego, School of Medicine, San Diego, CA, USA

Michael M. Talamantes University of Denver-Graduate School of Social Work, CO, USA

Mary R. Talen Resurrection Family Medicine Residency-AMITA Health, Chicago, IL, USA

Deborah A. Taylor Central Maine Family Medicine Residency, Lewiston, ME, USA

Ana Catalina Triana UCSF Faculty Development Fellowship, San Francisco, CA, USA

Aimee Burke Valeras NH Dartmouth Family Medicine Residency/Concord Hospital Family Health, Concord, NH, USA

Andrew S. Valeras NH Dartmouth Family Medicine Residency, Concord, NH, USA

Pamela Webber Fort Collins Family Medicine Residency, Fort Collins, CO, USA

Jackie Williams-Reade Loma Linda University, Loma Linda, CA, USA

Grace Pratt Integris Great Plains Family Medicine, Oklahoma City, OK, USA

Jonathan B. Wilson Crossover Health Medical Group, Dallas, TX, USA

Karen Wyatt Creative Healing, LLC, Silverthorne, CO, USA

Kat Gray Grand Junction, CO, USA

Artist Bios

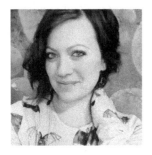

Kat Gray BS is currently a stay at home mother of two. She graduated from Colorado Mesa University with a bachelors degree in psychology in 2011. Kat had focused her love of art and psychology together while working as the activities coordinator at West Springs Psychiatric Hospital for six years before starting a family with her husband. Outside of caring for her children and home, Kat enjoys painting, drawing, baking with her children, and tribal belly dance. Her artwork is found on pages 70, 263, 277, 292.

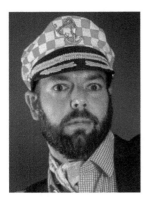

Luke Woody is an illustrator, designer and creative director from Austin, Texas. With pen, ink and other media, he distills complex themes into simple, striking visual stories. His artwork is found on page 139.

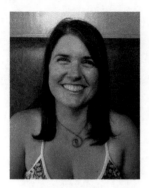

Sabrina Motta RN BSN is a school nurse with Mesa Valley School District 51, previously employed by St. Mary's Family Medicine Residency as a triage nurse. Her background in medicine started as a reservist and volunteer firefighter EMT-Intermediate with Durango Fire and Rescue. Outside of her career in medicine she works as a freelance artist and enjoys mountain biking, swimming, skiing, camping, and rafting with her family. Her artwork is found on pages 44, 95, 140, 194, 250, 296.

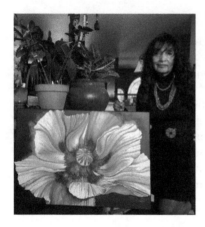

Yvette Campbell is a painter, hiker, and biker who lives in Grand Junction, Colorado. Her artwork is found on page 268.

Family of Origin

Electronic supplementary material The online version of this chapter (https://doi.org/10.1007/978-3-030-46274-1_1) contains supplementary material, which is available to authorized users.

Aunt Peg

Colleen T. Fogarty

The taciturn aunt,
      no children of her own

Taught me pie-baking
      when I was young.

Once, I bumped the tin
Berries scattered everywhere.
A scolding; No pie for me

Tears started—
Wait....

Gathering the berries, she gently washed them,
Helped re-shape the dough.

A vivid lesson—
perseverance, second chances,
      and even—
         the importance of forgiveness.

Different Fathers. Different Sons.

John G. Spangler

The photo is old and yellowing, curling at the edges, crinkled across Kodachrome color.

It's 1962.

You are in sky blue overalls with a white shirt and white, toddler shoes. You sit on your weary father's lap. He is beginning to bald and wears tortoise rimmed glasses, so much younger than you ever remember.

You are facing him. He is falling asleep, tired after a long shift as a third-year radiology resident.

This is the first father and son photograph you knew. You did not know him well in those early days of residency, and the first years of junior partner at the community hospital in your hometown.

Even in middle school, your days began at 6:00 am, swim practice or splitting wood; his days started with an early intravenous pyelogram. You did not enter his world often, and in those days, he rarely entered yours.

He was always on call, you see. With only 1 phone line at home, and no beepers back then, the phone was off limits with the exception of a 1-minute rule. "If you *must* make plans, go ahead." But a minute is not long enough for friends or plans or dreams.

Sometimes, if you were lucky, you would ride with him on Saturdays to the hospital and explore as he read out weekend films: The Wards, The 1-room Emergency Room, and The Door to the Morgue. At least, as the youngest, you had these special times with him.

So at a young age, you could discern the right and left hemidiaphragm, recognize a thyroid scan with a cold nodule, "diagnose" a broken bone—which he sometimes asked you to do.

Looking at a radiograph together, he would say, "What do you think is wrong with this leg?" The compound fracture would be obvious, even to you.

At home, you had scalpels, and syringes, and sutures and needle holders for sewing up a slit orange, or a ripped blanket. You had a chemistry set.

He brought home lead containers for you that had held radioisotopes at the

> You must understand, your mother counsels. Doctors were different back then. Unquestioned. Life was dribbled out by him to you. You pretty much just had to accept that as your filial duty.

Department of Radiology. You melted these down over a homemade Bunsen burner and spilled liquid metal into cold water to make wonderful, globular creations as the lead instantaneously re-solidified.

He placed radiation in tumors. Today, you wonder having been exposed to radiation residue and leaden fumes.

You dream at that age that you will be a physician, just like him.

As you progressed through college and medical school, somehow you could relate better to him. He understood straight A's, $1.00 apiece. He understood Phi Beta Kappa, a $500 reward. As you began to grasp his world, you could share these single things together, like a conversation.

Late one night during your own residency, in the dark corridors of Johns Hopkins Hospital L&D, your own son is born. You saw many births at the county hospital as a third-year medical student. You delivered them yourself at that impressionable age.

You are accustomed to the acral cyanosis of those first moments that flush pink with the lusty cry of full newborn lungs, shaking off the shunting, shutting off the ductus.

But this birth is different. The doctor hands you your 6-minute-old son, Apgars 8 and 9. He has big, black searching eyes, as if he is scrutinizing your face.

He has your hooked big toes.

Your firstborn son! The night passes like a dream.

He's 1 of 6 of your brood of children. You enter their lives with gusto, as if to compensate for your own childhood.

You take call nights and do diapers. Discharge patients and rush home to help with dinner, bath, and bed. Every chance you can—you live 5 blocks away—you hurry back for lunch.

Is it for you? Your wife? Your own youth set ajar? Or for your 6 that you lunge your whole being into their lives like your father could barely dip his big toe into yours? You must understand, your mother counsels. Doctors were different back then. Unquestioned. Life was dribbled out by him to you. You pretty much just had to accept that as your filial duty.

Yes, Sir, Lieutenant!

But times change, and with this different time come different fathers.

Preparing for boards last month, your son with your toes came home for the last few days of STEP 1 study. You quizzed him on Roth spots and Koplik spots and Rocky Mountain Fever spots.

You didn't remember the classes of antiarrhythmic medications. But your Apgars 8-and-9 son does—which he explained to you carefully and mechanistically and in detail the indications, contraindications, and side effects.

And tonight is his first night on call as a third-year medical student.

He texts you:

Him: *Peds neuro 6 wk old late onset meningitis Group b strep*
You: *Recent cheese outbreak here Listeria*
Him: *Rx that with ampicillin*

Of course, he knows that. You smile.

You: *Yep good luck tonight love you*
Him: *Love you too*

You know he is well on his way.

Cat Stevens laments in *Father and Son*: "I was once like you are now, and I know that it's not easy to be calm when you know something's going on."

Your father was once like you. And you were once like your son.

But you are different fathers, and you are different sons—

Each with different dreams, yet each with the same old, new perspectives.

Donuts in the Cemetery

Alexandra Schmidt Hulst

Touchdown in Dallas. The familiar overhead ding sounds and passengers lurch into the aisles, stretching and yawning and clamoring off the plane into a muggy Texas September afternoon. I breathe in slowly, gather my bags, and quickly shed my fleece sweater. My husband of 4 months squeezes my hand as we exit the airport, giving me a small, reassuring smile.

An hour later, we walk in the door of my grandparents' house, and I think "I am home" as I inhale the familiar smells of 65 years of raising 9 children, cooking for family, and countless dogs. As I quickly gaze out at the lawn and around the familiar hallways of this old house, I think of spring mornings searching for Easter eggs with my cousins, lazy rainy afternoons watching squirrels scurry through the ancient trees, and jam packed Thanksgiving dinners full of boisterous laughter and football blaring from the den. "Deep breath," I think to myself, swallowing down sadness as a quick round of hugs begins. Family has arrived from Atlanta and Boulder and Cedar Rapids as we prepare to say goodbye to my grandmother on this Labor Day weekend. Though the house is full of people, it feels more empty without her here.

Click clack. The slow sound of shoes stepping gingerly across the tile floor of my grandparents' church. More hugs, more family arriving for the visitation and the rosary. My husband whispers to me, "Do you think you'll cry tonight seeing her?" I shake my head naively, thinking that it won't feel real that she's gone until I see her casket being laid in the ground. As I think of how her lungs used to torment her as she gasped for air in the final months, I whisper back, "We saw her 3 weeks ago. I said what I needed to then. I'll be ok. I'm thankful she's not suffering anymore." He gives me a quiet look of I-know-you're-wrong-but-I-won't-say-it. Wise husband.

Seeing my grandmother's face—so familiar and so foreign—in the casket does bring me to tears, surprisingly and not surprisingly. More powerful than this is the way my heart simultaneously breaks and heals by watching my family grieve: quiet sobs, heaving shoulders, stifled sniffles, tight embraces, sad smiles shared across the aisle. I think to myself, "I love these people. My people."

The next day, we celebrate a funeral Mass for Shirley Marie Uhrik. Mother of 9. Wife to Richard Uhrik for 63 years. We sing How Great Thou Art, we soberly file out of the church, and we drive over in a long line to the cemetery. The priest joins us at the gravesite as we squeeze in together under the tent, trying to escape the blistering sun. The prayers, accompanied by a somber bagpiper, feel familiar from my childhood and evoke quiet sadness and reflection.

The rest of the burial though is filled with much more laughter than any of us expected. The releasing of the doves somehow goes terribly wrong; rather than all the doves being released into the sky in one beautiful move, they anxiously slip out of the basket one by one and hide away in a nearby tree. The newly minted dove trainer looks sheepish when he is scolded by the black-suited funeral director and apologizes endlessly. We shrug our shoulders and joke, "Grandpa and Uncle David are just playing tricks on her to welcome her into heaven." Even in our sadness, we can laugh and give grace to others.

Even more unexpectedly, the vault has not been installed into the ground. The funeral director seems very distraught by this and anxiously offers to have us come back in an hour or two when they are finished, but my family sees it as a chance to spend an extra hour with my grandmother before she's lowered into the ground. "We'll stay," we quietly decide together and settle into our chairs. Whether it's to keep a somber vigil with her one last time or make sure she doesn't come back to haunt us, half buried, is anyone's guess. The Irish are a superstitious people; we won't take any chances on an unfinished burial.

As we watch her grave being prepared, my uncles tell mischievous stories that would make my grandmother groan in her grave. They share with us out-of-towners their small act of rebellion. When my grandparents were planning their funerals years before, my grandfather wanted a bagpiper at his funeral, but when the time came to bury him, my grandmother refused since she thought it was tacky. Now that my uncles were planning her funeral, they decided to "forget" that little detail and hire the bagpiper anyways, just for a little lighthearted spite. "She's Irish…surely she wants the bagpiper but just didn't know it." So many irreverent jokes: something about the casket swinging open and her falling out. The rest of us shake our heads, pretending to be annoyed, but we laugh. "Tamp it down! Make sure she can't get out," one of them calls out to rings of laughter from the group.

Suddenly, I feel a flash of slight embarrassment, thinking of the strangeness of this entire moment and prepare to apologize quietly to my husband, so new to my family's antics. You can really only know the depths of how embarrassing your family might be when there's a new observer. But then I notice his grin, his quiet banter, and his recognition that the family needs this relief amidst the sorrow. He's one of us now.

Over the next hour, we curiously watch the mystery of a burial stripped away. It seems so unholy to have a close-up view of the workers in their stiff gray uniforms, the heavy construction machinery, and the dump truck filled with dirt. All these are the parts families are typically sheltered from so they can focus on the emotions of grief. I think of the appalled look my grandmother would have on her face if she could see all this going on, but the rest of us seem to enjoy the way watching these pragmatic tasks gives a bit of a needed break from the heaviness of death. This seems appropriate; my family has always vacillated between facing emotion head-on and having tough conversations and shying away from things that seem too painful to talk about, whether it was about dementia or alcohol abuse or depression or dying or faith. Or maybe, because my grandfather was the epitome of an electrical engineer, we've all inherited a fascination with how anything and everything gets done.

As we watch the dirt layer over this deep hole in the ground where my grand-mother will stay after we leave and return home, my husband whispers to me, "How do you want to remember her?" It takes me longer than it should to answer with a simple shrug, but tears slide down my cheeks. Right now, I don't know how I want to remember her. All I can remember of her at this moment is an oxygen concentrator and labored breathing and weak muscles that kept her homebound and visiting my grandpa at a memory care unit before he died. But I know that if I think deeply, there was a time that they were both healthy and fully alive: holding hands and squabbling and hugging grand-kids and walking through the alley to get to the hidden creek. I think of my grandpa tinkering with the garden in the backyard, smelling like wild garlic and onions, and my grandma sitting at the kitchen table chatting, one leg lazily crossed over the other. These are the memories that are both hard to summon and hard to forget.

> The next day, I wake up to the sound of rowdy laughter in my grandmother's kitchen. I hear familiar voices and join them. "Want to come with us to the cemetery?" my uncle asks. "We're going to have donuts and chocolate milk and visit Grandma."

The next day, I wake up to the sound of rowdy laughter in my grandmother's kitchen. I hear familiar voices and join them. "Want to come with us to the cemetery?" my uncle asks. "We're going to have donuts and chocolate milk and visit Grandma." As if this were a totally normal thing, I say, "Sure!" and head back to invite my husband to join us. "We're going…where? To do what?" It was then that I realized this probably needs some explaining.

As many families do, my grandparents had a long-standing tradition of going to the cemetery to visit loved ones who had died. It was especially important to them to visit loved ones who had died in World War I and World War II, not wanting their sacrifice to feel forgotten. Somewhere along the way, donuts and chocolate milk got added into the equation. No one really knows the exact origin of why: maybe remnants of an old Midwest ritual, maybe bribery for young children to go visit long-gone ancestors, maybe a nod to the banquet feast of the afterlife?

Now, 50 years later, this is still a way my family remembers those who have died and gives us a place to go relive all the tales that families love to tell. In all the years I've been making donut visits to the cemetery with the family, it's never been a very serious affair. There is usually laughter and storytelling and little bits of sadness and reality—they're gone, really gone, and all we can do is visit them here—scattered throughout, but not so much that an observer would probably notice them. You really have to look for the seriousness, but it's there, kind of like sprinkles on a donut.

Family-of-Origin: Things Aren't Always What They Seem

Julia Sager[1]

I am on a flight to Tucson, cruising at 36,000 feet above sea level, thinking to myself how extremely lucky I am that I don't succumb to flight sickness and usually am able to use plane flights to get a lot of work done. Not this time. My sister, who is across the aisle from me, sits up suddenly screaming, "He is poisoning me," and starts unbuckling her seatbelt. I fear that she is going to try to flee. After desperately not feeding into my own fears about what else I will uncover, I ask about her fears, unsuccessfully redirecting her. I guide us on breathing skills that we had practiced the day before, which proves to be unsuccessful. She starts escalating, "He has hidden cameras hooked up all around the house. They are connected to the locker room in the local gym, where they are all watching me." This is hour 5 of 9 of our travel. Thank God for the lovely flight attendant, who is more successful in redirecting my sister's emotions and focus. I am completely drained and realize that I will need to constantly engage my sister, for the rest of the day.

My goal is to stabilize and support her while we travel across country to one of the top inpatient rehabilitation programs for persons with comorbid mental health and substance use disorders. I will be dropping her off at midnight, where she will be involuntarily committed. This is number 5 of what will be 8 mental health hospital commitments for the year.

I flash back to my junior year in college, when I arrive home with my boyfriend for spring break on a Sunday evening, asking, "Where's Mom?" upon finding my father sitting alone watching television.

---

[1]Published anonymously under a pen-name.

He flatly informs us that, "She is in the loony bin," after which he immediately returns to watching his program. I am dumbstruck. Mom had never exhibited any symptoms of mental illness. I am filled with shock, sadness, and finally anger at my father.

Why didn't anyone tell me about this? How can dad be so disconnected? Is mom safe? I am enraged that he tries to forbid my siblings and me to visit her while she is hospitalized. For the remainder of my week home, my father refuses to discuss the matter, to visit my mom, and goes to work as if nothing has happened. I find out what

> He flatly informs us that, "She is in the loony bin," after which he immediately returns to watching his program.

had happened to my mother from my younger brother. I have to see that she is safe. My brother and I visit her in the hospital and she is discharged home 5 days later. She will spend the next 10 years suffering on and off psychosis.

This spring break week during my junior year was when I started questioning my assumptions that had led me to want to pursue a career in counseling. Up until that fateful week, I had thought that my family had given me the values and resources that aligned with the "helping" professions. We were financially "well-off", were weekly church goers, and were even the default church choir. My 4 siblings and I sat in a middle pew every Sunday, singing loudly, gladly, and in five-part harmony. I come from a large Irish Catholic family, with my mother always telling us that "everyone wanted to be like our family." We were fun, "normal", and had lots of love and warmth. I had bought into this ethos. Thinking that I had been given so much, I thought a life purpose of giving back would be a life worth living. I hadn't been conscious of the other "gifts" my family had given me. Not until my late teens did I start realizing that our family struggles were pretty atypical.

On a deep, internal level I had learned how to survive, if not thrive, in a very complex, chaotic family where tempers raged, drinking was often over-the-top, and emotional issues were acted out or brushed under the rug. I was the fourth child, but my needs were often fifth as my parents struggled to raise 2 children with emergent bipolar disorder and another with ADHD. I frequently felt unheard and occasionally unsafe. At age 6, I remember thinking, "Why would my 11-year-old brother lock me in the closet for what to me seemed like hours and not get in trouble?" At age 8, I thought, "When I grow up I will never live in this town, as much of what goes on is not good for me and seems really unhealthy." At 12, I remember seeing the chaos of my family through the shock in the eyes of my best friend as she witnessed some of the injustices. *Maybe my family dynamics aren't so "normal."* Upon returning home from a date on my 21st birthday, I thought it bizarre that my parents and older brother had "gifted" me one of my brother's friends, passed out drunk, blabbering incoherently underneath the family pool table. They thought this was hilarious. *How in the world do they think that this is so funny? What do I do with my disgust and outrage with this?*

My mother's initial psychotic break occurred 6 months later, which caused the ice to crack in the glistening surface image that she had painted and I had accepted about the ethos of my family. To dive below the surface and put the broken pieces together, I eventually sought out therapy. How I chose to be understood was to have a wonderful group of close friends. How I chose to be heard and recognized was to do really well academically and in the community. I was extremely active, sought out, and accepted leadership positions in sports, student council, and almost anything that might legitimately get me out of the house and away from our family dinners. I would avoid the family drama and get my accolades outside, rather than inside, the home. I learned how to keep my nose to the grindstone and keep moving forward in the midst of the chaos around me.

I still think that my family is lots of fun, has lots of love, and has contributed much to why I became a therapist. Although I have always been able to chart a straight course while "all hell is breaking loose", I work to be in touch with what lies beneath. I am pained by the shortcomings of our mental health system that does not always do a great job in balancing harm to self and others versus self-determination for persons with mental health or substance use disorders. I have experienced the importance of clinical advocacy and see the need for political advocacy for this population.

Ultimately, my sister stabilized after much advocacy, family support, and eventually initiating monthly intravenous anti-psychotics. She is now doing better than she has in years, if not decades. My mother stabilized and during the final 20 years of her life returned to being the warm, emotionally engaging, and supportive woman she had always been. I understand how my father's embarrassment, shame, and stigma about behavioral health issues played out constructively and not so constructively in our family. I never did talk with my father about how he dealt with his anger during my mother's illness. He had a stroke, developed expressive aphasia and eventual dementia at about the time when I could have processed this with him.

Now that I am past the age when my mother exhibited her initial bipolar symptoms, I am thankful that neither I nor my children have exhibited such symptoms. I am thankful that I have chosen a loving, emotionally grounded husband, and we have not replicated my family of origin's patterns of reacting to emotional pain and mental illness. I have learned some of my potential blind spots and have worked to change how I dealt with conflict as a child… earned respectfully and proudly within my family of origin. I embrace being in touch with my patients', my family's, and my own full range of emotions from gratitude to anger and judgment.

I know that my family of origin experiences help me to assist others to constructively respond versus react to their ostensibly dangerous, unwanted emotions. I can also help them become conscious of and deal constructively with their reactions, understanding the potential for shame, guilt, and sadness. I am grateful for my connection to family and the lessons learned. I remind myself daily that how we present ourselves may not always represent what lies beneath.

Where's Taffy?

Deborah Taylor

At 2 years of age, just 9 short months after being adopted by Terry and Ralph, I was diagnosed with osteosarcoma. The abnormality was first identified by a local newspaper photographer who took my picture for a birthday celebration. An astute local pediatrician in a small town in Maine facilitated our expedient connection with Boston Children's Hospital in the fall of 1958 that resulted in the devastating diagnosis. This account is told from the prespective of my mother's loving voice in my head...

You were admitted to Division 28—a large one-room ward at Children's Hospital with 14 cribs down each side. The unit was for children under the age of 5 from all over the world who had been diagnosed and were being treated for various types of cancers. I stayed with you while your father remained in Maine to work and financially support the family. I was sustained by a younger sister who provided daily hospital transport along with an evening meal and a lot of support. You "lived" in the hospital for over a year, requiring multiple surgeries and extensive radiation. The doctors, along with the rest of our family's healthcare team, became an integral part of your adopted family. We were blessed to have Dr. Midas as your oncologic surgeon. During your treatment course, I taught and reminded you of the story of King Midas and how everything he touched turned to "gold". Your Midas was a female surgeon who always offered the "gold-standard" of medical care.

As you neared the end of the hospitalized part of your recovery, your father and I, along with your care team, began to see some light at the end of the tunnel with the goal of returning to Maine to re-establish our family at home again. You had endured a lot (multiple surgeries and toxic levels of radiation therapy) yet consistently showed a spirit of determination and resolve. We defined you as a "little girl with a big attitude and britches to match." You frequently resisted help, and insisted on being your own boss—we came to describe that as your "adopted only-child rearing up".

One morning, your condition began to precipitously worsen—your prior spirit and resilience took a dramatic turn downward. You reported not feeling well but could not really identify more specifics to me or your healthcare team. An extensive workup failed to identify a cause. I remember the significant concern on Dr. Midas's face as your presentation worsened over a 48 hour period—you refusing to eat or get up and move around. Dr. Midas pressed me to consider if there were any factors that I was aware of that might be tapping your life spirit. I, too, was baffled by your deteriorating health. Dr. Midas made frequent trips to see you over that time and became more frustrated that the team, led by her, was ineffective in helping you rally.

> Taffy was a scruffy yellow stuffed cat that had been your only possession at the time of your adoption.

"Where's Taffy?" you said in a most irritated voice at Dr. Midas's first visit of Day 2. I recollected that we locked eyes and both immediately knew at the purest gut level that this could be the key that would unlock the mystery of declining health. Taffy was a scruffy yellow stuffed cat that had been your only possession at the time of your adoption; while I cannot tell you from where he originally came, I do know that he had traveled from the orphanage in southern Maine up to home in central Maine and then to Boston for your cancer care stay. He never left your side. He was with you going into surgeries, traveled to the daily radiation treatments, slept with you, ate with you.

Dr. Midas and I went into hunt mode—scouring your bed and the area around it. Dr. Midas called for your nurse to see what she knew. No one had seen Taffy for a while and no one could guess how long. Dr. Midas, however, knew exactly for how long—just over 48 hours—that is how long!

Taking matters into her own hands, Dr. Midas headed straight to the hospital laundry and reported later that she had the entire laundry team looking for Taffy. He was found in about 15 minutes, having weathered a washing and drying likely wrapped in your daily changed bedsheets. Scruffier than ever, he landed back in your bed. I remember the look on your face when you saw him—the glee, the giggles, the hugging, and refusal to let him go for any reason. Over the next few hours, you began to rally. Within a 12 hour period, your health had re-stabilized to its previously good status—good energy, no complaints, eating well, back to saying no, resisting help, and being feisty. Taffy was home again and you were well again.

I have heard my mother tell this story many times. I have learned a lot from many valuable life experiences, but no lesson more powerful than the one this story conveys. It has helped to drive me to attend to those less tangible factors that can heavily influence and alter health and well-being. It informed my choice to pursue a doctoral degree in health psychology and then spend 3 decades as a family medicine educator. My mission has been twofold: (1) To help patients understand the value of giving voice and power to those powerful yet often intangible influences on health, and (2) to help medical students and family medicine residents understand and appreciate the value of attending to the whole person in the context of their life and its important influences. I have found that we all seem to have one or more Taffys in our lives—the relationships or stories that can build or destroy health.

The Resilience of a Child

Michelle K. Keating

In medical school and residency, you always heard about the resilience of a child. I believed it, but I wasn't quite sure what it meant. I had seen children quickly recover from severe bouts of croup or a 24-week preemie breathe on his own for the first time. But, I still didn't *know*. That is, until I experienced it with my own child.

My daughter, Abby, was 2 years and 3 months old to the day. She had the most beautiful, long brown hair, that she constantly wanted braided to be like Doc McStuffins. She stated with conviction that she wanted to be "a doctor like Mommy" since 18 months old. However, for a few months, she was more tired and clingy than usual, battling some weird symptoms—random bouts of vomiting, diarrhea, recurrent infections—that I couldn't put together.

She developed a painless limp. I turned to my husband nearly in tears, "Ty, I think Abby has leukemia." His response wasn't quite what I expected. "Michelle, you have to stop playing doctor-mom and just be mom!" He was frustrated as he had put up with a few months of my incessant worrying about our child. We discussed it further and both agreed to take her to her family doctor.

In spite of her near-normal blood counts 3 weeks earlier, my colleague examined her and agreed to re-draw a CBC. I canceled the rest of my day and brought my precious child home to snuggle with her, before trading off to my husband to go back to work for a late meeting. In the middle of my meeting, my colleague called me. She never called, she always texted. I silenced it and sent her a text, "In a meeting, do I need to step out?" She immediately replied with one word, "Yes." My heart sunk. I stepped out into the hallway by my office and called her. "Michelle, Abby's white count is 40,000." I dropped to my knees and bawled, "Abby has leukemia."

All of my medical training didn't prepare me for the whirlwind that happened next. We arrived at the pediatric emergency room at the hospital where I had been trained, now working, and where she would ultimately receive all of her treatment. I had never seen this side of it. We repeated blood work and Abby had to have additional X-rays. She wanted her mommy, but her daddy had to accompany her to X-ray because I was 26 weeks pregnant with her baby sister. She was overwhelmed, but Ty and I kept telling each other, nearly constantly, "We have to hold it together for Abby." My instinct was to do a PubMed search on childhood leukemia, but my wise husband forbade me and insisted I focus my attention on being *Mom*.

> As a mother, it broke my heart to allow them to pump these toxins into her little body, but as a physician, I knew this was what was required to keep our sweet baby alive.

Abby had Acute Myeloid Leukemia (AML). *Cancer.* Every inch of my being aches with that word in the same sentence as my baby girl. We discussed the next steps with her pediatric oncologist, a colleague of mine. She would need a central line, lumbar puncture with chemotherapy into her spinal fluid, and bone marrow aspirate. Soon after, we were headed downstairs to the pediatric operating room and I handed my innocent child off to the anesthesiologists. Her treatment had begun. Without her dad or me there, she would receive her first dose of chemotherapy. As a mother, it broke my heart to allow them to pump these toxins into her little body, but as a physician, I knew this was what was required to keep our sweet baby alive.

The next 4 months were a blur. Her treatment consisted of 4 rounds of inpatient treatment with each round expected to average 21 to 35 days with a 7- to 10-day break at home in between. However, Abby had other plans as she astounded us with her longest hospitalization being just 22 days. Very early on, we were told she would likely have fevers and probably even a PICU stay, but we were determined to not allow that to happen. We had to be in near isolation during this time due to her weakened immune system as this doctor-mommy was not allowing anyone who had even the slightest sign of illness near her.

Inevitably, her course of treatment was not without complications. She lost a significant amount of weight and required an NG tube to give all of her nutrition through tube feeds. She developed fevers and required antibiotics. She required multiple platelet and blood transfusions. However, at one point, Abby was running the halls of the oncology unit wearing her favorite hat of the day, her bright pink N-99 children's mask, tutu, and "Anna and Elsa" slippers. One of her oncologists stopped us, "Did anyone tell Abby that she has leukemia?" It was great to see glimpses of our happy, sweet child back. By the end of the first round, her sweet, long, brown hair was coming out in chunks and breaking my heart with each strand that I pulled off me. But Abby didn't care, she would just tell me, "Don't cry Mommy. It's okay, it will grow back!" How was a 2-year-old comforting ME during this time?

Other times were extremely tough. One day, in particular, stands out. Her NG tube cracked and required replacement, followed by multiple X-rays in which she screamed and cried as her pregnant mommy could not be in the room with her. This felt like the ultimate form of torture as I cried, squatting outside the door to her hospital room. However, I've never been more thankful for an incidental finding on X-rays. They found she had pneumotosis intestinalis—air and inflammation in her gut wall—a very dangerous complication of one of the chemotherapy drugs she received. She was placed on gut rest, started on IV antibiotics, and required around-the-clock fluids. She could not eat or drink for 6 days and then was allowed to slowly drink 5 teaspoons of Pedialyte and eat 5 Cheerios until she was tolerating foods again.

Throughout her treatment, Abby spent 83 days in the hospital. She received 82 doses of chemotherapy, 5 blood transfusions, 7 platelet transfusions, 3 bone marrow aspirates, 4 lumbar punctures, 2 feeding tubes, and 1 central line placement. She had 3 echocardiograms, 8 X-rays, went under anesthesia 6 times, and had to have 30–40 dressing changes for her central line and feeding tube. Despite having no immune system for almost 4 months, she did not succumb to a single viral infection or require a single day in the PICU.

Knowing what we know now, Abby had a relatively easy treatment course compared to other children who battle AML, and for that we are extremely grateful. However, like all childhood cancer survivors, her course will never be completely over. She requires frequent checkups and blood work for the next 5 years before she can be considered cured. We have to monitor her heart closely because of the chemotherapy she received. She has to be revaccinated for all of her childhood vaccines, which has been the hardest part of the course according to Abby! She is at risk for developing other cancers and we can't be sure if she will be able to have children in the future.

As I sit here on the anniversary of her diagnosis, I now *know* how resilient a child can be. My daughter is living proof of it. From just sitting there calmly with her mask on while the nurses changed her dressings to running the halls full of energy when her hemoglobin was so low that she required transfusion. We call her our warrior princess and she is that and oh-so much more. And, at the end of all of this—hospitalizations, pokes, imaging, being away from home—Abby still says that she would like to be a "doctor like Mommy" when she grows up. My child is the definition of resilience.

My Father's Death and My Own

Paul D. Simmons

From my father, I learned: Compassion. Unwavering adherence to decisions, once he'd reached them. Indifference to superficial honors. Hard work. Persistence.

—Marcus Aurelius

My father, born to a cotton sharecropper in rural Texas in 1939, is dying. He has widespread, metastatic liver cancer. They teach us early in medical school to deal with death at a psychological distance. Within days of starting my first year, I was cutting into the leathery, embalmed body of a petite, 73-year-old woman to learn anatomy. Even her thin, delicate hands, the most psychologically challenging part of her to dissect, eventually became metacarpals, extensor tendons, and branches of the radial nerve. Her body became a tool for my education. A tool deserving respect and gratitude, certainly, but nevertheless a tool.

But to hear one's own father has nodules in his lungs, a large mass in his liver, and to know what that means, collapses the carefully constructed psychological distance. The tissues and anatomic structures so painstakingly learned are suddenly irrelevant.

I am walking the emotional tightrope of being both physician and son. I am not my dad's doctor, of course, but still may be the doctor he trusts most, and the family depends on me to interpret treatment plans and prognostications. At the same time, I am losing my dad, and despite my love of science, statistics, and evidence, I am surprised to find myself more afraid, more bereft, and less able to "be objective" (whatever that means in this situation) than I'd hoped. I keep finding unrealistic hope in the next round of chemo, hope that I wouldn't find based on the evidence alone if he were any other patient in the same situation. Strangely enough, he may be the most realistic one in our entire family.

It is not everywhere that death shows himself so near at hand; yet everywhere he is near at hand.

—Seneca the Younger

We human beings, like all living things, are destined to die. It seems we are the only animal that knows we will die, and everything we do is shaped by that knowledge. When a parent dies, it means we children are next in line. My mother, most likely, will die next, but loss of parents means loss of a shield of sorts between our generation and death. My brother, the oldest of 3, will likely come next, followed by my sister, then I will die. Of course, this order is merely probable—with death there are no guarantees other than its inevitability. Now that dad is dying, I will not only face his mortality, I am facing my own. Is what I've accomplished so far in life worthwhile? Do I want to spend the rest of my life the same way? What will I leave behind, if anything?

> I am losing my dad, and despite my love of science, statistics, and evidence, I am surprised to find myself more afraid, more bereft, and less able to "be objective" (whatever that means in this situation) than I'd hoped.

These reflections have filled the last two months since Dad's diagnosis confirmed his mortality. I've been telling myself that my experience is not unique—everyone's parents die. I have taken comfort in the fact that—unlike too many children—I've had a wonderful, present father who loved my mother throughout a long marriage.

My dad is not perfect by any means. He carried on the racism of his Southern upbringing, using the "N-word" in jokes until his children told him that his grandchildren would not grow up around that word. He taught me several lessons about women that I had to unlearn as an adult after repetitive bad relationships. I've always wondered if he's proud of me, if I am "man enough" to earn his respect even though I cannot fix a car or build a toolshed. And I've too often taken the lazy, easy route of blaming him for my own failings as a man.

I don't believe that I will ever see dad again after he dies. Many believe in an afterlife, including most of my own family, but I do not, so I can't seek comfort there. Instead, I do take comfort in his life which, as far as I know, was well-lived. He rose well above the poverty into which he was born, and made the world a little better for his being here. I take comfort that he still has his mind intact, and that we as a family have a few months to have those last conversations, to hear his memories, and to say goodbye.

Let us strip death of its strangeness; let us spend time with it, let us get used to it, let us have nothing on our minds more often.

—Michel de Montaigne

Life is full of tragedy. If we do not have something terribly wrong with us or someone we love right now, we will. And beyond the tragedy, there is malevolence—people, some of whom we love, will hurt and betray us. How do we deal with the darkness? In the end (so to speak) it comes down, I think, to an individual choice. The choice is always ours: do we judge reality as unjust and flawed, slipping to impotent rage or nihilism when hurt by life? Or can we manage to bear the inevitable tragedy and pain with courage, selflessness, and maybe even love? Maybe that's the only thing that can justify our flawed existence, after all.

Dad has faced his end with courage and selflessness, indeed. He has talked more about not burdening the rest of us with his "arrangements" than about his own suffering. He speaks about how my mother is taken care of, has a paid-off home, and will be okay. I believe he is proud to have left the world 3 successful, contributing children, and several grandchildren.

He is giving his body to the local university to be dissected by a young medical student, like I was, who will use his body as a tool to learn anatomy. And will learn from my Dad's hands—those skilled, calloused, loving hands—the bones, tendons, and nerves he or she will need to know. If that's not bearing suffering with nobility and love, I cannot imagine what is.

Real Doctor

Laurie C. Ivey

"Why don't you be a real doctor," he said, as we discussed my career aspirations. Images of his discontent flashed through my mind, in addition to the gut crushing insult. Why would I want to follow in his footsteps? He might be a prestigious physician, but he's also a drunk. Wait, that's a secret!

I felt a chasm of disconnect with him. The last thing I wanted to do was be anything like him, but I had his body, the exact shape of his calves, his build, his genes.

I feared my destiny would be misery and discontent, too. However, I was very motivated not to let that happen. I had my eye on being a psychologist, which would ensure a better outcome.

He died in the middle of my graduate school applications, the day before I was scheduled to take the Psychology Graduate Record Exam. He and my mother had started to enjoy partial retirement. He had worked hard to reach this point and was allowing himself some recreational pleasures. I was in the midst of my post-college launch—college degree in hand, working in a coffee shop, before Starbucks ever left Seattle.

I experienced more relief than grief at the time. His death meant no more egg-shells or fear of alcoholic rants. It meant freedom for my mother from this trauma. It meant freedom for me from his judgments. It also meant I didn't have to tell him I was gay.

I moved to Denver for my doctoral degree in Clinical Psychology. I worked hard to get as much clinical experience as possible, particularly in working with people who experienced trauma—sexual assault, domestic violence, burns, veterans, torture, and war trauma. After working with torture survivors, my level of vicarious trauma peaked and I was screaming in my sleep, just like the victims of torture with whom I was working. When the faculty behavioral health position opened, I applied and got the chance to work in primary care.

I was apprehensive about working in a primary care practice, wondering if I was walking into a job full of "my fathers." I feared that the medical providers would be close-minded, conservative, critical people who hated and looked down on psychologists. I encountered a couple of residents like this early on, but that was the exception and those two wandered off to specialty residencies. Instead, I discovered amazing professionals who worked hard like I had done, because they wanted to make an impact on others. They were smart, quick-witted, engaging, and loved to banter. They certainly didn't always know what to do with me. In fact, when I started my job, I met with my boss and asked him what he wanted from me. He shrugged, hands out, palms up, and said, "I don't know, you figure it out." That was ok with me.

> I would have urged him to get a primary care doctor. As I rolled out our wellness curriculum, I often felt sad that this was not a part of his training.

I felt a strange sense of reassurance with my new home in family medicine, as I had felt having a doctor as a father. Growing up, my concept of home wasn't always psychologically safe, but I knew my father was smart and if someone was sick, he could fix them. He had this reputation in our small town. He was the town "Doc". He was revered.

Despite my faith in his medical acumen, he wasn't always tuned into my illnesses or his own. He ignored my childhood bout of pneumonia for 2 weeks and felt ashamed when he realized this. He was not tuned into his own physical problems or mood problems. He had no personal physician to help him identify his struggle with alcohol, depression, and stress. He never connected the impact of these factors on his health. His undiagnosed heart disease led to a massive heart attack at age 61 killing him almost instantly. Despite these misgivings, I always respected his knowledge and maintained faith that doctors know and heal all.

In my new family medicine home, at age 30, I also started learning about and grieving the connection that I could have had with my dad had he not died an early death. I would have called him up and enjoyed telling him that I spent my afternoon teaching his types about my world, via didactics on treating people with depression or perhaps personality disorders. Maybe, I would have shared a couple of examples to encourage him to try and heal. I would have urged him to get a primary care doctor. As I rolled out our wellness curriculum, I often felt sad that this was not a part of his training.

Many days as I drove home, I thought about how I would have told my dad that a physician handed her patient off to me today to help the patient manage her panic symptoms after a trip to the emergency department the night before.

I thought about how I would have been excited to have him teach me about the vasovagal response and its physiology. I know I would have endured endless complaints about changes in the business of medicine, and eye-rolls and expletives about the emergence of the electronic health record. I would have loved to discuss opinions on health care for all, and try to sway his lean to the left.

I've questioned what force plopped me into a career in family medicine. I certainly believe it was not by chance. It was to help me understand the parent that I most struggled to understand. It was a chance to attempt to grieve. I am left with a deep longing for the conversations that I didn't get to have. It is a regret and a loss. It is also likely a continued search for fatherly approval. I hope from somewhere out there in the universe, I am getting at least a partial nod.

The Cigarette

Karen Wyatt

One of the most reliable tools I've used in my medical practice is story—listening to and sharing the tales of life to help patients heal their old narratives and begin a new chapter that offers more promise and more potential for creativity. But I have sometimes found, in the midst of retelling a patient's story, that I have also healed parts of my own broken narrative at the same time.

My father first inspired me to become a "story-gatherer" with the imaginative yarns he would spin while we sat around the campfire during family fishing trips. He talked of his uncle Bob, a sheepherder who taught him survival skills in the Bighorn Mountains of Wyoming, and a mysterious character he called "Slats" who lived by the railroad tracks and showed him the secrets of successful fly-fishing on the Middle Fork of the Powder River. Dad would regale us for hours with suspenseful tales of encounters with rattlesnakes, mountain lions, bull elk, and grizzly bears from which he had narrowly escaped during his adventures in the mountains. Through Dad's campfire tales, I learned the art of deep listening so I wouldn't miss a single detail that had been woven into the fabric of the story.

It was no surprise that, with the influence of my father, I came to see the entire world around me as a series of fascinating stories unfolding before my eyes. Even when I worked as a bartender to support myself in graduate school, I fell in love with my job because it enabled me to listen to stories all night long. To me, life has always been a perpetually spinning narrative with heroes and villains, plot twists, impossible predicaments, turning points, miraculous resolutions, and a well-defined beginning, middle, and end.

My story-gathering ability proved to be quite useful when I began my career in medicine. My technique involved speaking less and listening more deeply so I might discover a key detail that would lead directly to a diagnosis or treatment plan. Sometimes, I worked with patients who were frustrated because they had become stuck in the middle of their own life stories and couldn't figure out how to get to the next chapter. My job was to help them navigate through a difficult plot twist in order to get the story moving forward once again and my motto became, "The answer is in the story ... just listen."

In one case, a 36-year-old woman named Jill came for her first visit with me because she wanted to stop smoking. The story she presented was that she had tried to quit for the past 2 years and had exhausted every option available. I was the most recent of a dozen professionals she had consulted for help and none of their recommendations had worked for more than a few weeks. She had used patches, gum, medications, hypnosis, acupressure, yoga, meditation, psychotherapy, prayer, aerobic exercise, fasting, and various herbs—all to no avail. Jill told me she no longer got any pleasure from smoking so she couldn't understand why it was so difficult to give up. She was miserably stuck in the middle of this story of hers and saw no way to shift the narrative.

> When her stepfather yelled at her or punished her, she would thrust her hand into her pocket, feel the cigarette there, and regain the determination she needed to survive his emotional attacks.

While Jill carefully recited her recollections of every failed remedy she had tried, I recognized that there was a different story that needed to be told. So I asked her to share with me when and why she had first started to smoke—and that's when things got interesting.

Jill began to describe how her mother had raised her alone after her father abandoned them when she was 5 years old. She remembered being very happy until age 14 when her mother remarried a man with 3 younger children. Suddenly, her entire world was disrupted. She was forced to move across town, change schools, and adjust to her mother's new relationship and expanded parental duties. The 3 younger children demanded a huge amount of her mother's time and Jill was often left to fend for herself.

Her new stepfather was a strict disciplinarian who imposed rigid rules on the household and saw Jill as an annoyance. Having moved away from her old friends, she started hanging out with a rough crowd at her new school who encouraged her to try smoking. Jill said that when she took her first puff of a cigarette, she hated the taste but loved what it represented. Smoking made her feel strong and confident because she was defying her stepfather's rules and was being her own person.

And then Jill revealed that she used to carry a single cigarette in her pocket at all times to remind her of her strength and independence. When her stepfather yelled at her or punished her, she would thrust her hand into her pocket, feel the cigarette there, and regain the determination she needed to survive his emotional attacks.

As I listened to Jill describe her loneliness and despair during those teenage years, the deep story behind her smoking history became obvious to me. "The cigarette was your best friend," I told her. "Smoking helped you survive a difficult time in life so it's hard now to let it go."

"Yes," she agreed, "that's what I feel each time I try to quit smoking ... like someone I love has died."

She realized that her emotional pain had driven her back to the cigarette over and over again. A war had been raging within her between her teenage self who clung to smoking as an important part of her identity and her adult self who was repulsed by the habit and wanted to be free of it.

The next chapter of Jill's story—the resolution of her narrative arc—became clear as we spoke together. I told her that the cigarette was not the villain of the story but a supporting character who had played a pivotal role in her development. I suggested that she stop trying to eliminate smoking from her life and instead begin to carry a single cigarette in her pocket just as she had done as a teenager. In this way, she could still keep close her "best friend" that had once helped her survive. The presence of the cigarette would also soothe her fear of losing her independence and identity when she was ready to give up smoking altogether.

Before she left, she told me that no one had ever asked her to tell that story and she seemed relieved to have released an old memory. I never saw Jill in the office again after that day but 3 months later, she called to say that she had not smoked since our visit together and she was still carrying a single cigarette in her pocket every day. She wondered why it had been so easy to stop smoking this time and I told her simply, "You healed your story."

I was pleased to learn that our interaction had been helpful to Jill, but somehow I had not been able to get her story and the image of that cigarette in her pocket out of my thoughts. I didn't understand why but a familiar pain from my own unspoken story would rise within me each time I thought of that cigarette safely tucked away.

My hidden story was of my father's suicide that had taken place several years earlier and had left me on my own to try to weave together the loose threads of his raveled narrative—the ultimate challenge for a story-gatherer. At the time he made the decision to end his life, he had recently retired from his work at the gas station he inherited from his father. For months he had been complaining of insomnia and vague anxiety that constantly haunted him. He didn't understand where those feelings were coming from but as a survivor of many treacherous adventures, he believed he could find his way out of this situation, that he would discover his narrow escape; and I believed it, too. Ultimately though, he found an escape route that brought an untimely end to his story and completely disrupted my own. Dad was the hero of all of my childhood memories—he wasn't supposed to die by his own hand.

The pain I carried after his death was so devastating to me that for years I couldn't bear to talk about it to anyone—not even my mother and brother. I was afraid to speak of the overwhelming guilt I experienced as a doctor trained in behavioral health who couldn't save her own father from suicide. Those feelings had remained deeply buried for years until the cigarette in Jill's pocket brought them to the surface for some inexplicable reason.

Then one day many months later, I received an insight that provided a clue to this mystery. My brother and I were having lunch together when he took his wallet from his pocket and along with it came a grimy, well-worn rabbit's foot. He reminded me that this was the very rabbit's foot our father had carried in his pocket throughout his service during World War II and every day until his death. Though dad would not talk about the details of his combat experiences, he did share that he believed his lucky rabbit's foot kept him alive and got him through the horrors of war, much like Jill's cigarette had helped her get through her challenges earlier in life.

The rabbit's foot in Dad's pocket was a symbol for the stories he could not tell: the trauma he had experienced in war and his guilt for having done harm to others. Perhaps, his hidden stories were a clue to his suicide, though I will never know the answer to that question. But I could see that the story of Jill's cigarette had served as a trigger for this memory of dad and a pathway into my own untold story of guilt and pain over his death.

The stories we keep hidden have the power to change our lives for better or worse. As practitioners, we become skilled at helping our patients retrieve those stories and rewrite them to tie together the loose ends of life. But sometimes, there is a perfect twist in the plot when the teacher is revealed to be the student after all. At the intersection of our stories of pain, there is an opportunity for both lives to begin the process of healing and resolution. And sometimes, all it takes to open that door is the simplest detail, like 1 ordinary cigarette tucked away in a pocket.

Holding Hands

Pamela Webber

Last night I took a picture of my aging parents, holding hands as they dozed on the couch. Mom and dad have always been hand-holders, in private and in public, while walking, chatting, and eating; they have held hands. I remember once, years ago, my daughter found it frustrating that they held hands on a busy sidewalk in Dublin, slowly navigating the crowd as a pair instead of single file. This simple physical connection that my mom has to my dad is one of the few things that have not deteriorated since her diagnosis.

My mom has Alzheimer's disease. This is a reality that my family has been dealing with for 5 years. Into her 70s, my mom stayed active with travel, volunteer projects, and social activities. A diagnosis of Alzheimer's was not a certainty but also not unexpected; my mom had seen the disease in her own mother and knew that 3 maternal aunts had also been diagnosed with Alzheimer's dementia. She and my dad were so excited when, early on in this journey, she had neuropsych testing and was told that she had "mild cognitive impairment," but not Alzheimer's disease. As a family physician, I could see that the deficits she demonstrated during testing pointed to early Alzheimer's. I have often wondered if my mother also knew but concealed many of her struggles during these early years. When the official diagnosis finally came, I was amazed at how openly my parents shared with friends and family, even announcing it in their yearly Christmas card.

The disease progressed as time passed, but my parents were able to compensate until Mom's memory and Dad's poor hearing caused communication challenges. I found myself using my communications training learned both as a family physician and marriage and family therapist to facilitate some difficult conversations. As Mom's memory and executive skills decreased, my father took a more active role in managing the house. The former director of the public library system, my father was accepting, positive, and calm in the face of adversity. When mom expressed that she regretted not being able to do things for dad, he told her, "You took care of me for 55 years, now it is my turn." Mom stopped cooking, then driving, then volunteering. By June of 2015 they took their last big trip, a birthday trip to Hawaii with my sister and her husband.

The following year brought more decline. Mom lost weight and lost interest in activities; she slept most of the time. I started coming over almost every night to cook dinner; she seemed to eat better when I cooked. She developed shingles, which I hoped to be the cause of these new symptoms, but she did not improve as expected. Our family and her physician attributed her symptoms to her dementia and dad started the process of hiring caregivers for some respite during the week.

Then one Saturday, my dad called and told me that mom was in severe pain. I came over, put a hand on her abdomen, felt how tense it was, and told him that we needed to go to the Emergency Department. There, the nurse palpated her abdomen and pointendly asked if I had felt the mass. My immediate thought was "No, I missed it." But, that initial thought was replaced with what really happened: in my role as daughter, coming to my parents' aid, I had done nothing more than a superficial exam and rushed my mom to the ED. I had not palpated my mom's abdomen. I have long accepted the role of medical expert in my family, as I am the only trained medical professional, but I have always refused to do anything very involved. Diagnosing shingles after looking at the area where my mom was complaining of pain was one thing, but palpating my mom's abdomen was crossing the line I had drawn between daughter and doctor.

The ED physician ordered a CT scan and the final diagnosis was gallbladder cancer, with a prognosis of less than 6 months to live. Masked by the dementia, her pain and the cancer had been stealing her appetite and her energy. We were offered 3 choices: a biopsy to confirm the diagnosis, a procedure to decompress the gall-bladder, or no procedures at all. Dad chose the third option—no invasive procedures. Mom was hospitalized for 2 nights to ensure that she had good pain control, offered regardless of which option we chose. Dad spent 2 nights in the hospital in an uncomfortable pullout bed. "She saved me," he had told me, "so now I am going to be there for her." He shared that he was on a self-destructive path when he met my mom and because of her influence he completed his education and became a professional and a family man. This was not the end-of-life path he had anticipated. His parents died before age 65, while my mother's parents lived into their 80s. She was supposed to long outlive him.

Mom was discharged to their 100-year-old home, now in chaos as an electrician had been hired to rewire the whole house. We sat in an upstairs bedroom and mom, holding dad's hand, struggled to relay important details of her past. She wanted us to remember that she preached an Easter Sunrise Service at Red Rocks Amphitheater as the president of the Colorado Council of Churches; to know where she put the items she gathered for her memorial service. She made it clear that she knew that she had cancer and would probably die soon. My dad and I reassured her that we remembered these details. At the same time we worked on the practicalities of calling hospice and home health services, somewhat relieved that she might not suffer the long slow course of Alzheimer's disease.

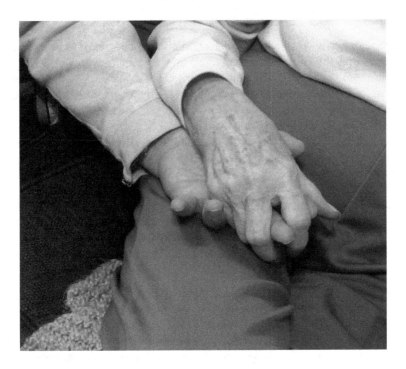

Eventually, my mom's pain was controlled, the family had rallied, and home health and hospice were going smoothly. Mom was eating better but was still very thin and frail. In a few months, my sister from Alaska and my brother from Pennsylvania arranged to be in town at the same time so we could take a family picture. We did the same thing, decades prior, 3 months before my mom's father's death from cancer. My dad appreciated this chance for a final family portrait. I saw my parents' acceptance and adjustment to their new end of life path, and gratitude for the visits they received from friends and family during this time.

Then, the end did not come. Life surprised us, and it continued. For days, then weeks, then months, then seasons, my mom made a comeback, her appetite and activity improving. After 9 months on hospice, she was discharged. We are now 3 years out from the cancer diagnosis and 6-month-life-expectancy prognosis. My mom's physical health is better than when she received the terminal diagnosis. Progression of her cancer seems to have slowed but sadly and as anticipated, the mental deterioration from Alzheimer's disease continued. Just as my family rallied around the cancer diagnosis, we are now settling into the unknown and pro-tracted course of Alzheimer's dementia. For the family in town (my dad, brother, and me) that course is long and wearing. I have continued to work full time and struggle with the balance of patient care, teaching, time with my parents, needs of my adult children, and self-care. When the diagnosis was cancer with death imminent I comfortably could ask for flexibility at work. It has become much more difficult to ask for or expect that flexibility as time passes.

Even though her physical health is better, Mom continues to deteriorate. One of the things that the caregivers asked when they first started coming was, "What did your mom like to do?" The only answer I could come up with was "plan and organize." How do you organize when you have Alzheimer's disease? Mom folded and refolded the blankets on the couch. Now there is less of that. Mom used to get frustrated and worried that dad would leave her; some days she was certain that he had taken all of their money and had a girlfriend. The ability to verbally express those fears has been lost. She used to enjoy visits from family and friends but more recently has become agitated with the change in routine that comes with having guests. The most notable decline has been in language and communication. Mom will often start a sentence, "Do you want..." and trail off into silence. I have gotten very good at non-answers and model them for my family, "No, I do not want anything," or, "I have everything I need right now." This same technique comes in handy when she is anxious. "Dad and I have taken care of it," I will assure her, whatever *it* might be.

My image of Alzheimer's disease has been shattered by my mom's course. I hoped she would be pleasantly demented, and that we would be able to share in some charmed reality created by her mind. Instead, her inability to communicate has created a place that I cannot go. So, we experience being lost together and I find myself talking, giving hugs, and sitting close. Just as the Alzheimer's has slowed her, it has slowed and refocused me. It has allowed space to reflect on this strong, assertive woman who supported my dad in his work and her 4 children in their various activities. She was my role model in following my educational dreams, inspired me to accomplish projects and taught me how to navigate the world as a strong woman. The cancer diagnosis did not spare her, or my family, from her continued decline. Now together we explore the world of *not being able to do*—her because of the Alzheimer's disease and me, because despite my medical and therapy training, there is nothing I can do.

Through all of this I see my parents taking each day as it comes, laughing when they can and celebrating their time together. About a year ago mom started telling people that "she was supposed to die but is still here." As her family we told her that, "we are glad you are still here." She started to express that she felt like she needed to be in a nursing home. I told her that we "would look into it," though we had no intention to do that. Even now, my dad and I should probably be looking into it, but he is committed to having her at home. With 2 supportive children in town and the financial resources to afford caregivers, he can make this decision and continue to hold her hand in their home while they fall asleep on the couch watching television.

My Fathers, My Family

Randall Reitz

My 3 earliest memories are of my dads.

At 3 years-old, I went out for burgers with my young mother and brother. The street-side burger stand had a treehouse with a slide that I loved. We kept an extra chocolate shake in a blue patterned cup for my father, Paul, who was propped up against pillows at home. He smiled and embraced us, struggled through the shake, and vomited it on his pajamas and sheets.

My second earliest memory is of staring into his casket at our Mormon chapel. I wanted to touch his face with my little-boy fingers, but worried that it was inappropriate to touch the dead. My grandmother watched me for a second, came to my side, and in her queer way, asked me, "Do you know who that is?" Of course, I did. She tried to comfort me: "He's in heaven now, and no longer in pain. You'll be there with him, too, some day."

My third memory is perching on my soon-to-be new dad's shoulders as we walked by Christmas displays. I was the third-wheel on their first date. His shoulders were broad and tall and I could tell they looked comforting to my mom also. This was 5 months after my first memory and 4 months after my second.

Just like these 3 memories, I'm sure this narrative has inaccuracies and gaps. Childhood memories are easily elaborated, as are the memories of people facing death and living beyond the death of loved ones. The moral of my narrative is that death destroyed my family, death created my new family, and death forever shaped me and my career.

***

Dave and Shawna were high school sweethearts who married 2 years after graduation and lived in a mortuary to save on rent as they raised their boys. Dave worked full-time as a veterinary lab tech while he studied microbiology at the university.

About 3 years into the marriage, Shawna went to bed with flu-like symptoms, awoke past midnight, and collapsed on the bathroom floor. Hearing the thump, Dave ran to her side, assessed her, called 9-1-1, and started CPR. She was declared dead moments after the ambulance sirens quieted. No one knows the exact cause of her death, but we suspect it was congestive heart failure caused by a virus.

> Throughout the years of my personal and professional life, I've come to appreciate the rare gift of my father's death. Not that he died and I lost the opportunity of knowing him, but the way he died and how my mother was supported by family and our community.

Dave is a responsible man who is known for preparation and stoicism—both of which were overwhelmed by this sudden loss. He soldiered on through the funeral, but then reality set in. He had sacrificed time at home so he could work and study. Now he needed to add single father, cook, and cleaner to his roles. While he was sustained by his faith and the support of family, he distinctly recalls an exhausted body, frantic mind, and his own collapse to the bathroom floor, in a fit of despair.

My first memory of Dave is of Christmas lights and strong shoulders, but I imagine that exhaustion and despair also accompanied him on his first date with my widowed mother. The deaths of their spouses occurred 9 days apart. While they hadn't met before being set up on a blind date, they somehow had 3 friends in common, none of whom knew each other, but all of whom were independently convinced that their meeting needed to happen. These friends saw parallels in their lives and hoped that a strong family could be forged from their shared losses.

While there are similarities in their stories, the years have allowed my mom's marriage to Paul and his premature death to take on a heroic arc, whereas Shawna's loss still feels tragic.

Mom had known for a while that something was amiss with Paul's body, but for months, his rare Ewing sarcoma had been misdiagnosed as a foot fungus. Once accurately diagnosed and aware of his poor prognosis, he continued working and participating in outpatient radiation and chemotherapy in the evenings.

Paul, like Dave, demonstrated quiet fortitude, so mom was surprised when she attended his treatment for the first time and was informed that Paul only had a few weeks left to live. This was before the hospice and palliative care movements, so they cobbled together in-home care with a neighbor who was an RN and a family friend who was a phlebotomist—the same friend who lined up mom and Dave for their first date.

Throughout the years of my personal and professional life, I've come to appreciate the rare gift of my father's death. Not that he died and I lost the opportunity of knowing him, but the way he died and how my mother was supported by family and our community. Family was with mom when Paul drew his last breath at home and has been unfailing in support throughout my life.

In a recent email, mom described the struggles of these early months: "After it was all over I became pretty angry. We had already lost a little girl. He was a good man, we had just finished grad school 3 years before and he'd lived a healthy life. My boys needed a dad and I needed a husband. I decided I had 2 choices, I could either let it get me down and be bitter and angry or I could rise above it and be a better stronger person. In his death, there was no middle road."

Bringing together their families was not an easy task. I've wondered whether it was initially a marriage of convenience—focused on meeting the basic needs of Maslow's Hierarchy. But, I believe them when they tell me that romance and shared experience was what brought them together. Their song has always been Debbie Boone's "You Light Up My Life." Their love lit up their lives and their faith carried them through the hard times of the early years to where they are now: happily retired, the parents of 7 children and 23 grandchildren.

Along the way, our family has endured many difficult illnesses. My youngest brother, Chad, was diagnosed with diabetes at age 8. My sister and sister-in-law have MS. My daughter suffers seizures from epilepsy. There have been many, many pregnancies, not all of which have gone smoothly or resulted in healthy children.

This intimacy with illness and death focuses my mind. My experience with dead parents embodies my work with families. How is my patient holding up? Who is supporting her? Who is supporting her supporters and providing respite? How can we shore up this family in distress? What are the beliefs, strengths, and resources we can rally to their cause? How can we approach their remaining days so they reflect the strength of the prime of their lives, rather than the sterility of their final surroundings?

It would surely be easier to only focus on the person sitting next to me in the exam room and to ignore her family and community, but Paul and Shawna, and Nancy and Dave, require more of me.

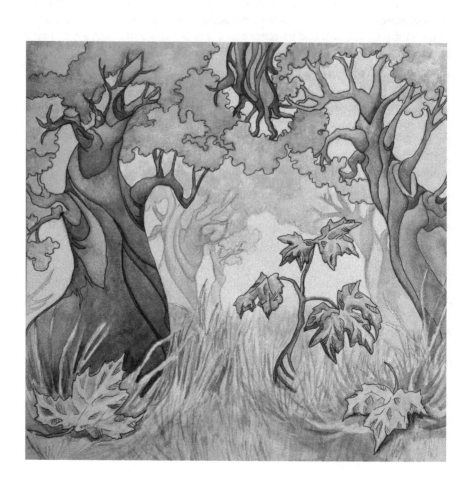

Reflection on Family of Origin: Grow Up and Leaf Out

Juli Larsen

Sitting on the ground, with our back up against the rough bark of a beautiful maple tree, we gaze up through the branches and green canopy to the sunlight above. The sun filters through the shifting forms of the leaves, dancing around the seed pods that hang delicately from the branches. We watch as the wind drifts through the seed pod cluster, and one pod slips from its mooring, softly falling toward the earth.

Our gaze follows the seed pod as the wind lifts under its long slender wings and carries it across the field to find its final rest in the undisturbed earth, far from its family tree. We begin to consider the unique attributes that the seed pod carries within it, attributes that will allow it to grow into a beautiful maple tree. We also consider the environment that this seed pod finds itself in - drier, more exposed than the family tree, and we wonder if this small seed pod knows how to adapt in order to thrive.

Imagine this seed pod sinking into the ground, finding root, sending up a shoot, leafing out, and beginning its growth cycle. Much of what it does, it does because it is programmed by nature; however, there comes a time when out of necessity, this young tree will fine-tune its functions, allowing it to fully develop and grow.

Imagine watching as this young tree engineers the bark that surrounds and protects its core, developing the precise rigidity to yield to the wind without breaking. Taking a cue from the dry earth, the roots sink deeper into the ground, bringing nourishment and life up into the canopy. The leaves miraculously open and close small pores releasing or retaining the right amount of moisture to allow for health and growth.

All of this is done to the unique specifications of the tree and its environment. The tree adapts for optimal growth. It is a beautiful miracle.

Just as miraculous and noble, is the development of human beings, not just in the physical realm, but extending into all realms. Our DNA may set in motion our physical development, but our imprints set in motion our emotional and relational development.

These imprints come from our home environment, boundaries, and nurturing that we received from our family. Sometimes these influences are a blessing to us, other times they are a detriment. Shifting to these balanced views, and updating unbalanced views, allows us to develop relational and emotional skills within ourselves and others.

In life, however, we often don't make deliberate choices, but fall into reflexive choosing based on our imprints.

Consider that somewhere, in our emotional scaffolding, we may have a belief that we need to be perceived as sufficient in order to be accepted. With this belief we may reflexively choose to hold back and refrain from risk taking, fearful of falling short of the mark. In so doing, we limit our opportunities for growth. Without examining these unconscious beliefs and allowing them to inform our deliberate choices, we cannot develop the necessary and unique characteristics that will allow us to fully grow and mature. Reflexive choosing hinders our ability to assess what our true needs are and adjust our choices to meet those needs.

Though some of our internal scripts feel intuitive, creating this reflexive choosing, the various environments we find ourselves in invite a continuous examination of these scripts. We assess if they are congruent with the environment and the growth we wish to achieve in that setting. In this process, like the tree, we are figuratively choosing how far our roots will sink and in what directions. How thick our bark should be and how we will leaf out. We update our imprints in an effort to influence our deliberate choices that lead to growth.

This is the process of self-development. When we fall into reflexive choice, we often try to manipulate our environment, including relationships and situations, in order to fit them within our limited abilities to adapt. Either the environment has to change or we have to change. We often perceive it to be easier to change the environment than ourselves. Just like a tree, we cannot control the harshness of the wind or the depth of the water. Often, all we can do is adapt to the environment in which we find ourselves.

Adaptability is the rule of nature, and so it is with the human experience. We bring goodness into the world as we choose those behaviors that allow us to grow up and leaf out.

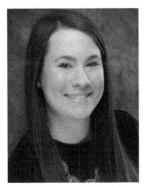

Alexandra Schmidt Hulst PhD, LMFT is a medical family therapist who has had the honor of working alongside incredible team members in primary care, a pediatric intensive care unit, and an adult neuromuscular clinic. Her first book, titled Contextual Therapy for Family Health: Clinical Applications, was published in 2018. She lives in Grand Junction, CO with her husband, her son, and her pup; they are her biggest fans and best inspiration.

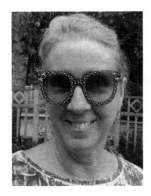

Julia Sager MSW, (pen name) has a long history of behavioral science teaching. She currently consults on behavioral health, curriculum design and team development for multiple medical and non-profit organizations. She is passionate about keeping humanity and relationship sacred in primary care. When not consulting, Julia designs and models innovative eyeglass-wear, illuminating the world view and faces of those who wear them.

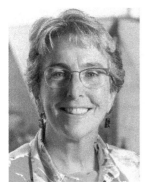

Deborah Taylor PhD, died On October 6, 2021. She had a long and distinguished career as behavioral science faculty at Central Maine Medical Center's Family Medicine Residency. She was a beloved mentor to dozens of early career behavioral science faculty around the United States. We are honored to include her story, "Where's Taffy?" in our book.

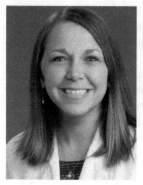

Michelle K. Keating DO, MEd, is an assistant professor at the Wake Forest School of Medicine and Wake Forest Family Medicine Residency. She Received her Bachelor's Degree in Chemistry from Kalamazoo College, her Doctor of Osteopathic Medicine from the Edward Via College of Osteopathic Medicine-Virginia Campus, and her Masters Degree in Health Professions Education from Johns Hopkins University. She has a passion for evidence-based medicine, medical education, and humanism in medicine. She loves to spend time with her family, traveling, and finding the joy in every day life.

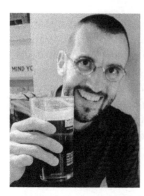

Paul D. Simmons MD, is a faculty physician at the St Mary's Family Medicine Residency. He received his bachelor's degree in History from Baylor University in 1995, and his medical doctorate from the University of Colorado School of Medicine in 1999. After several years of practice in rural settings, he has been teaching residents since 2010. Outside of work, he enjoys CrossFit, trail running, obstacle course racing, Stoic philosophy, and his pets—all of which are impermanent.

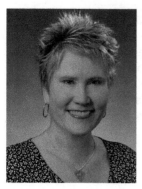

Laurie C. Ivey PsyD, is the Director of Behavioral Health at Swedish Family Medicine in Littleton, CO and is the Director of their Integrated Primary Care Post-doctoral Fellowship Program. A clinical psychologist by education, she has been training Family Medicine residents for 16.5 years and has been training psychologists in the field of integrated primary care since its early beginnings.

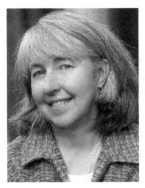

Karen Wyatt MD, is a retired family medicine and hospice physician. She graduated from the University of New Mexico School of Medicine and completed Family Practice Residency and a Fellowship in Psychiatry at the University of Utah. She has written extensively about end-of-life care, including the book What Really Matters: 7 Lessons for Living from the Stories of the Dying. She hosts the popular podcast End-of-Life University and is passionate about helping people find meaning and purpose even during the most difficult times of life.

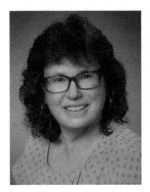

Pamela Webber MD, LMFT, is Associate Director of Behavioral Health at the Fort Collins Family Medicine Residency Program in Fort Collins, Colorado. She completed her MD at the Universit of Colorado in 1990 and her MA in Marriage and Family Therapy at the University of Colorado in 2009. Outside of work she enjoys hiking, reading and spending tme with her cats, friends and family, including her parents.

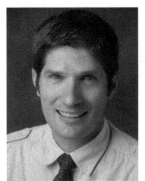

Randall Reitz PhD, LMFT, is the Director of Behavioral Medicine at the St. Mary's Family Medicine Residency in Grand Junction, Colorado. He completed his doctoral studies at Brigham Young University. Outside of work he enjoys trail running with his wife, mountain biking with his children, and baking with his thoughts.

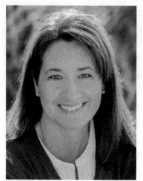

Juli Larsen BS, C-MI, is a meditation instructor in Grand Junction, CO. She completed her undergraduate work at Brigham Young University, majoring in Health Promotions. She enjoys philosophical conversations with her husband, discussing good books with her 5 children, and spending precious quiet time swimming and gardening.

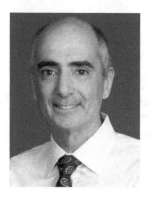

John Spangler MD, is a Professor of Family Medicine, Psychiatry and Epidemiology at Wake Forest School of Medicine. He has a strong interest in addiction medicine and obesity as well as the epidemiology, prevention and cessation of tobacco use. He leads two opioid addiction clinics and tobacco cessation group and individual counseling sessions. An avid writer, he has widely published in the medical literature and academic and lay press. His greatest passion is his family of six children and two grandchildren and he also enjoys reading and ethnic cooking.

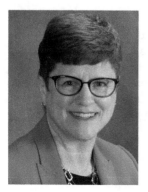

Colleen T. Fogarty MD, MSc, FAAFP, is the William Rocktaschel Professor and Chair of the Department of Family Medicine at the University of Rochester Department of Family Medicine. She earned her MD degree at the University of Connecticut School of Medicine in 1992. Dr. Fogarty is considered an expert in writing 55-word stories and using them as an educational tool for self-reflection. She has published many of these stories, poetry, and narrative essays in several journals.

Teachers and Mentors

Electronic supplementary material The online version of this chapter (https://doi.org/10.1007/978-3-030-46274-1_2) contains supplementary material, which is available to authorized users.

Wisdom from Mentors

Colleen T. Fogarty

By now you have entered your cave of fear

Wrote a beloved early mentor,
early in intern year.

You think too much; you talk too much

Said a visiting Tibetan Buddhist healer
His words gave me pause.

As mentor, I aim to listen, reflect—more than diagnose.

You know best what you need right now.

We Believe in Us

Cameron Froude

I hustled along the winding path through Boston's Theater District, an area known to locals as the Combat Zone. An ominous gray sky overlaid the setting sun. Burnt orange and butterscotch colored leaves swirled around me. The caustic wind, atypical for early November, promised a bitter winter ahead. I wrapped a scarf tighter around my broad shoulders. As a born and bred New Englander, I never wore a jacket. I barreled ahead, racing against the clock to arrive in time for my final appointment. Gloves were for the faint of heart.

Moments later, I turned the corner and careened into a metal shopping cart. It brimmed with tattered luggage, crushed metal cans, and holey blankets. Charya, a slight Cambodian woman, squatted at the base of the cart. She rearranged items in the undercarriage to make space for an empty milk jug. I expected that Charya would be farther in line at this time of day. My stomach knotted on her behalf. She wouldn't even make it to the entrance of the shelter before dark.

I placed the triple espresso with a splash of condensed milk next to her. "Iced coffee in the winter?" I jabbed. "I don't know how you do it, Ms. Charya."

She jumped to her feet. "Thank you, thank you. I need to be more awake! See how far back I am?" She took my hand and held it between hers. "Your hand, it is very cold."

When Charya and I met for counseling, we drank Cambodian coffee as a ritual that connected her to home and me to her. She drank it "strong and cold." Charya's health insurance lapsed last year, and we could no longer meet in the clinic. Shortly thereafter, Charya's apartment building burned to the ground, and she lost custody of her son, Chea. Without a home or a counseling center, Charya and I continued our conversations in the community.

Recently, our relationship centered on barista bartering. I brought her Americanized Cambodian coffee in exchange for a gem from her cart. Generally, Charya presented me with a packaged pastry, half-scratched lottery ticket, or a trinket from a place that held meaning for her.

"I wish I came here earlier," she remarked. She paused, "But then maybe I wouldn't see you, so I'm glad for that. Life is life." Before I could respond, Charya kneeled to rummage through a paper bag at her feet.

> Find the pockets of humility in our mental health system and do good work. Stand for something complex in this world.

I inhaled deeply, the warm taste of nicotine cut the biting air. A few doors down, a man with a salt-and-pepper beard screamed empty threats into the air between drags on his cigarette.

Charya slipped a crème colored paper into the pocket of my sweater. She took both of my hands and squeezed. Her toothless smile grew wide. "This is for you, from me and Chea."

Finally, I reached the stout brick building nestled between a check cashing and liquor store. The clinic was on the second floor. My eyes burned at the site of the candy colored flashing arrow pointing at the LIQUOR-LIQUOR-LIQUOR sign just above the building entrance. The irony of that sign, a microcosm for how we spin our wheels in this country, never escaped me. The impossibility of healing any-thing—bodies, minds, souls—in our sick environments rattled my insides. The familiar fist of uncertainty about my purpose as a healthcare provider formed in my chest. *What's the point?*

I paused across the street to say a pithy prayer. Actually, it wasn't as much a prayer as it was a plea. It had been a full moon, manic Friday at the clinic. The day had consisted of back-to-back appointments, a report to child protective services, and an involuntary psychiatric hospitalization.

Please, I thought, *make this appointment go smoothly*. Both for my morale and sanity, I needed the intake with Coretta Anderson to be straightforward—hook, line, and sinker.

I ushered Coretta from the white-walled waiting room through the concrete corridors to the bare bones bunker where healing should happen. I sat behind a squat, metal desk. Instead of using the dingy, torn fabric couch, Coretta sat across from me on a plastic folding chair. Unprompted, she explained, "Me and dirt. We don't get along too good."

The base of Coretta's nose, pinched by a pair of bejeweled reading glasses, poked out from above a stack of state required paperwork on my desk. Coretta darted her squinted hazel eyes around the room. She scoped every inch of her environment.

The overhead lights flickered. I began the therapy machinations: First, photocopy the insurance card. Next, review the consent for treatment form.

During my adolescence and young adulthood, I worked in many establishments designed to support and assist people with mental illness. These experiences indoctrinated me into the institution of mental health. By the time I graduated college, I was fully inculcated into the institution and had adopted the definitive jargon and unapologetic expertise of our profession. Individuals were their problems. We labeled people delusional, delayed, disabled. We pathologized relationships as codependent. We framed methods of coping as disordered. Patients believed that I could use my professional skills to discover the truth of their lives. I also believed it.

Coretta burned a hole in my head with her steely gaze.

I typed and typed and typed and typed. Just yesterday my boss chuckled, "when you're not doing paperwork, I welcome you to practice therapy."

After finishing the last intake form, I looked up from my computer.

We have about 10 minutes left. Where would you like to begin?

Coretta shook her head, bewildered. "I can't say what I need to say in 10 minutes. I thought you were here to help me. Never mind, just forget it!" She stood, scowled, and walked out into the cold night.

Dr. Johnson, my sage mentor, opened the door and extended her arms. Desperation was an uncomfortable vehicle for change. And, on that day I was the driver. I bear hugged her and she wrapped her arms tightly around me. She smelled faintly of incense and cigarette smoke, a familiar scent into which I collapsed.

"I can't do this anymore," I sighed. "I'm drowning."

"It's good you're here then," she whispered, rocking her feet back and forth.

I slumped into the plush, cozy chair. A night-light with a spinning shade left prints of dolphins dancing on the ceiling. I lost myself in the rhythm of the round and round. Dr. Johnson sat back and admired the ceiling alongside me.

"Those dolphins have danced like that for forty years," she said.

I smiled. "Just like you."

"Just like me," she said, shaking her head.

"How do you do it?" I asked. "How do you do it day after day?"

She paused. "I give people their due time. I listen hard and speak free from my heart."

She held my knees.

"You said you're drowning. Well, I'm here, throwing you a rope. It's not a clean, pretty rope, but it's a rope. How do you want to be remembered by those you serve?"

My eyes widened. I could not begin to know.

"Let's start from the beginning," she said gently. "Describe how you loved as a child."

"I cared for others and they cared for me."

"That's how I always knew you," Dr. Johnson said.

I racked my memory for the turning point when relationships became secondary to another agenda. As I moved ahead in life, I surrendered the power of relationships. What was the trump card, though? I thought aloud.

In high school, it was rubrics and grades. Later on, I prided myself on flawless chart audits. Just recently, I prioritized a completed intake packet over a human being. How can I get back to when it was simple?

Dr. Johnson walked to a bookshelf and retrieved a chunky hardcover. She handed it to me. I cracked the compilation of portraits, opening to a wrinkly Vietnamese woman with sparkly eyes and a long narrow mouth. I turned a couple of pages. Pasty skinned twin sisters pinky-swearing in a sun-splashed lavender field, their fingers covered in mud. I flipped to a man with a furrowed brow and weather-beaten face. His hazel eyes were barely visible beneath a frayed cowboy hat. I felt nostalgic on his behalf.

Dr. Johnson pulled my focus back. "These snapshots. What do they mean to you?"

I studied the picture. A colorful, beaded necklace encircled the cowboy's calloused fingers. *When he was a boy, how did he imagine his life unfolding? Did he envision himself there, on the other end of that lens, or was he destined for something else? How many years did he toil in the sun? Who was his first love? His confidante?*

"Reverence and curiosity," I responded.

Dr. Johnson folded her hands into a steeple and rested the point beneath her chin.

"That's your humane reaction to a face, a person," she said warmly. "Your pure response."

"What's happened to me?" I asked softly.

She searched for the words. And then, after a moment, said:

"Our field, mental health. We train young people to deny the complexity of humanity with thick books of diagnoses, measures of health and illness. We favor rigid definitions of normalcy outlined in a chart over the hard work of learning the stories behind people's wrinkles, the legacies informing their choices. Our responsibility is to care for people, families, communities. Find the pockets of humility in our mental health system and do good work. Stand for something complex in this world."

My mind raced at the implications of Dr. Johnson's words. Every experience, relationship, and memory was a pearl. Our work, then, was not to identify the bad ones and toss them aside or polish them shiny. Rather, we must marvel at each one and string a necklace worthy of our patients' necklines.

Dr. Johnson gazed out the window into the bleak charcoal sky. I'm sure it would snow tonight. I remembered her buoyed step and fresh face the first day we met. She looked older and wiser today. Gray strands of hair swirled into her black locks, which were pulled loosely in a bun. Dr. Johnson shook her head: "We are healers, and we are people. Where does that paradox leave us?"

I pictured Charya and me on the side of the road, exchanging dumpster fortunes for faux Cambodian coffee.

"With relationships," I responded.

"Those will anchor you," she replied. "But first the wounds need to heal."

"I'll heal them," I promised. "I'll be me."

She nodded. "Be you always."

Coretta answered after one ring.

"Hi, Coretta," I said quietly. "Remember me, we met for therapy."

Coretta sighed, sucked her teeth. "I don't remember therapy. I remember you on the computer and then me leaving."

My face burned. I held my heavy head in my hand. Coretta needed boundaries, hard lines. Not realness and vulnerability. I heard Dr. Johnson's words, *be you always*. Always. All ways. I breathed.

In lieu of a well-oiled story about Coretta as a sick patient and me as a healthy professional, I lived with uncertainty about our relationship. I sat with feelings that brought me closer and farther from Coretta and myself. I turned over ruthless and compassionate thoughts in my mind, breathing through their stark contrast. Finally, my heart broke the cage free and I said,

"Coretta, I'm sorry for being horrible to you. That day—many days actually—but that day in particular, I was struggling to do everything I thought I needed to do for everyone. Everyone but you, the most important person. All of it left me drowning, gasping for air and cruel. That's not me."

Something loosened in Coretta's voice. "Well can you promise me that this time you'll help, that you'll fix it?".

My heartstrings pulled in the direction of promising quick expertise. I recalled my commitment to realness. I needed the boundaries and hard lines now.

"I can't promise to fix it. I can promise that I'll listen, ask questions, and share myself with you. And with those ingredients, we'll learn about you, about us. We'll fix it together."

"Yeah, I like that, it's good. Kind of like a friend, but as a counselor," Coretta replied.

"Yes, it's kind of like that," I responded.

Coretta and I spent the first ten minutes of our second meeting in absolute silence. She sat forward and parted her lips. I leaned in, waiting for her words. The heater crackled. People shuffled in the hallway outside. She leaned back. We repeated this dance. I imagined the reams of books she could fill with the words trapped inside of her body, caught in her throat.

"Coretta," I breathed. "Sometimes starting with a ritual can be helpful."

She cocked her head and narrowed her eyes. "Like praying?"

I paused, considering this idea. "I would be honored to pray with you."

Coretta motioned for me to stand. She moved our chairs and sat cross-legged in the middle of the floor. I clasped my hands together and sat across from her, our knees barely touching. I channeled Dr. Johnson, trusting in our vision of unfiltered authenticity and human connection. Coretta enveloped my hands in hers. We closed our eyes.

"Just follow me," she said. "We'll start where it takes us."

Coretta started her mantra and then the words spilled out of my mouth as if I'd said them a thousand times. Within a few moments, I had entered Coretta's prayer completely. I rode the ripples of her chant, "om namah shivaya, om namah shivaya, om namah shivaya." I ebbed with the deep vibrations of her alto voice and flowed with the infinite loop of the prayer, "om namah shivaya, om namah shivaya, om namah shivaya." Our voices blended into a rhythmic tapestry.

The vibrations of our voices resonated in the caverns of my chest. My neck throbbed and forehead pulsated. I felt dizzy and exhausted. My body was not my own. Instead of pulling away, I delved into the experience. In the space between my mind and eye, I saw a trout swimming along a narrow stream. The sharp focus of the vision jarred me.

I followed the fish around a mossy bend, inviting further exploration. It guided me into a maelstrom of winds and torrential rain. The heavy clouds bore down close to the earth. The trout swam rapidly beneath the stream's current. It slipped between boulders and fluttered among tall weeds, leading me with hurried confidence. The trout flipped itself out from the water and into the sky. His slender body morphed into long roots and his tail blossomed into a tree trunk and leaves. Oversized ruby apples adorned the majestic tree. Two young girls emerged from the earth like flowers, their arms outstretched reaching for the apples.

Poof, the vision vanished.

Coretta's chanting slowed and her voice lowered. "Where did it take you?" she asked.

I squeezed my eyes shut, pulling energy deep into my mind.

Now was the time for me to emerge from the shadows, to disclose my experience to Coretta.

"Coretta, my body ached, I was dizzy and tired. I saw a trout with rainbow gills swimming down a cobalt river. He led me to an apple tree. What does this mean to you?"

I opened my eyes. Coretta's body trembled.

"Olivia, my sister, my love. She's gone. She died for me and now she's gone."

Once she blinked the first tear free, one hundred generations of despair fell from Coretta's eyes. She bent forward, pressing her palms against my knees. She sobbed and wailed. I rested my hands gently on her shoulders.

Memories of Olivia came in flashes. Coretta described Olivia begging to be hit, spitting in their stepfather's face. "He didn't even provoke her," Coretta explained. "She'd ask for it." She recalled Olivia slouched on a stoop with a needle protruding from her arm. She remembered Olivia's tattooed wrist, handing Coretta her meal out the drive-thru window. Coretta pictured her sister straddling the torn vinyl chair at the visiting room of the prison.

"She sacrificed herself for us," Coretta sighed.

The most difficult memories for Coretta were Olivia's final days. Coretta described her sister at the end, hollow and frail, mumbling in her sleep, "purple and pain, purple and pain, purple and pain." She couldn't make sense of the days before her sister's death.

"What memory of you and Olivia can you rest with between this week and next?," I asked.

Coretta crossed her hands and gazed at the floor. "The one of us under the apple tree," she said. "That's a nice, peaceful one."

I nodded. "Yes, yes it was."

I woke early the next morning and walked the steep jaunt to the Charles River. I sat on the edge of the dock and grazed the bottom of my sneakers over the water. The Boston skyline twinkled, promising a day of feverish activity. A handful of sailboats bobbed in the icy water.

I reached into my pocket and felt Charya's note. I pulled the creased paper from my pocket with a heavy heart. I hadn't seen Charya in over a week. I placed my finger on top of Chea's small thumbprint in the corner of the paper.

The last time I saw Chea he had just left for foster care. We were in Boston Common, sitting on the ground against a concrete water fountain. He was eating a neon razzle berry ice pop. I had left the markers at my office and only had a red pen. "That's good," he said. "Now I can draw a heart."

I unfolded the paper, soft with wear. A tangerine sun with long rays and blue puffy clouds filled the top half of the page. Stick figures of Chea and Charya dancing with grins ear to ear were in the middle. A canary yellow bird flew between them. Just above its wing, Chea wrote, "you," and drew an arrow toward the bird. In large black block letters, Charya wrote: "We believe in us!"

Belief in the power of relationships was a germane part of my identity as a child. After years of education, I evolved into someone who I didn't recognize. I created and recreated my identity as a healthcare provider by and for my patients. I embraced the endless nature of this dance—learning and unlearning, declaring and questioning, writing and erasing. The process is the product, which is often a blank page, a moment of silence, a shared prayer. It is in the precious moments of authentic connection where we finally realize our most honorable intention as healthcare providers: To bring the shadows of ourselves into the light as the ultimate sacrifice to our patients, who trust us as the keeper of their secrets.

In Celebration in Memorium

Jeffrey M. Ring

On the chilly morning of January 18, 2017, the Boston Globe announced the following:

"BUDMAN, Simon H. Of Newton Centre, age 70, died unexpectedly the previous Friday at Brigham & Women's Hospital. Dr. Budman was an internationally celebrated scientist, innovator and entrepreneur."

Simon Budman was my mentor.

I arrived in Boston in 1983 to begin my training as a clinical psychologist. I had the great fortune to land a part-time job interviewing patients before and after psychotherapy on a depression outcomes study at what was then the Harvard Community Health Plan. The office next to Fenway Park was a beehive of clinical research activity and innovation. I felt the creative energy in the office during my interview.

I was feeling rather overwhelmed and alone, having just moved from Berkeley to Boston, and the research team became my family. Dr. Budman took me under his wing. He instructed me in research, clinical interviewing, team collaboration, and writing for publication. He generously included me as a co-author on our research report (Budman et al. 1988). Part of my job was to review videotapes of group and individual therapy delivered by Dr. Budman. Through those observations I learned about brief treatment models, the importance of focusing on the patient's target complaints, and the essential contribution of empathy and a warm sense of humor to rapport building and improved outcomes. I easily recall his broad smile now as I write these lines.

During my time in Boston, Dr. Budman agreed to serve as my dissertation chair and our relationship deepened. When he underwent surgery for an unexpected aortic valve replacement, I sat with him in the hospital. This was indeed a strange shift of roles and relationship. Dr. Budman had already offered me so much in terms of learning and opportunity; it was an unexpected pleasure to be able to give something back, even as I fumbled for the "right" things to say to my teacher draped in a flimsy blue and white hospital gown.

Months later after he recovered, he asked me to serve as the videotape guy for his daughter's Bat Mitzvah, a job I totally botched, lost sleep over, and then worried about the implications for our relationship and for my doctoral thesis! In the end he was understanding and forgiving. Dr. Budman taught me and guided me throughout those years in graduate school, always demonstrating great interest in my overall wellness, life balance, and social connections.

> My daily work is influenced by the lessons I learned during my time with you. You and your teaching continue to live inside me.

I left Boston for the University of California San Francisco in 1986 to begin a minority clinical psychology internship and postdoc. Life got busy: two years in Spain, a teaching job back in Los Angeles, caring for and losing a close family member, marriage, and parenthood. I did not really look back.

On January 11, 2017, sitting in my office in Los Angeles, looking out over Griffith Park, I called Dr. Budman and he picked up the phone. I had a sudden urge to reach out. It had been over 30 years since our last conversation which took place at a farewell party that he and the research team hosted in my honor. I still wear and cherish the blue fish bowtie they presented to me as a gift.

"I am so happy to hear from you, Jeff. Of course I remember you...but may I ask why you are calling me now?"

"I feel a compelling need to express my gratitude to you, Sir. Your mentorship and teaching have marked my career. My daily work is influenced by the lessons I learned during my time with you. You and your teaching continue to live inside me. It is important to me that you understand how grateful I am for you and for our time together."

Our conversation was warm and tender. He filled me in on his work, his family, his Bat Mitzvah daughter now grown. I told him about my work in medical education and health care consulting, about my family and other pieces of my personal and professional trajectory. We excitedly discovered a number of shared areas of interest and agreed to have our work teams meet for a brainstorm session the following Tuesday to explore potential collaboration.

As I sat in my office on Thursday, January 12, the phone rang. Dr. Budman called to let me know that he had not been feeling well and that he would be entering the hospital the next day for a cardiac procedure. Our brainstorm meeting, he said, would have to be postponed. I let him know I was sending all good thoughts and prayers for the outcome of his procedure. I thanked him for his call. I wished Dr. Budman goodnight.

Reference

Budman, S. H., Demby, A., Redondo, J. P., Hannan, M., Feldstein, M., Ring, J., et al. (1988). Comparative outcome in time-limited individual and group psychotherapy. *International Journal of Group Psychotherapy, 38*(1), 63–86.

Sugar-Coated Bitter Pills

Ajantha Jayabarathan

Why do we believe in happily ever after? Why do we sugar-coat bitter pills? Why do we bubble wrap reality?

My story is about living past happily ever after, tasting the bitter pill and breaking through the bubble wrap to experience relationship with others.

I was born in India. My father was selected to train in Canada, and in 1969, my mother, sister, and I joined him. It seemed like a fairy tale to me and as the plane taxied onto a snow-covered runway; my four-year old mind thought that Canadian sand was as white as the people I saw.

I have vivid memories of seeing, hearing, smelling, and tasting much that was utterly foreign to me, just as I was foreign to those I met. I learned to speak English by watching Bugs Bunny on television. I developed my insatiable curiosity about space from witnessing the moon landing. I can still feel the burst of energetic agency that I felt in this new land, where people spoke in soft voices, greeted you with a smile and affirmed in kindergarten that you could be all that you dreamed. My imagination was watered by an unquenchable thirst for information. My fertile mind, seeded with ideas that took root, soon grew a multidimensional, inner universe, where all was possible.

We returned to India when the year ended. My inner world remained intact, nurtured by books that I read. But my day-to-day life in India paled in comparison to my rich, inner, worldview.

After all, I was a girl born into India in the 70s. I was quickly shown my place in society. Men were revered; their accomplishments celebrated; their ideas never challenged. My self-expression was contingent upon my ability to get along and please in the male-crafted world that I lived in. I felt fettered. I ceaselessly worried that I was a ship destined never to sail. I resigned myself to a life of convention, in which nothing would match my imagination.

Remarkably, we were given the opportunity to return to Canada. Memories and dreams filled my sails as we journeyed back to the magical land that had long captivated me.

But the land I thought I knew so well was foreign to me once again. As I navigated through the loneliness and isolation of being a "very Indian 17 year-old" within a race of beautiful, vibrant, self-assured youth, the magic held within my mind

> When we align our ego and efforts with our inner pilot light, we are rewarded with insight, wisdom, compassion, empathy, love and peace.

continued to cushion me. They were kind and respected my scholastic ability. In math class, I would outdo them using Clarke's tables while they used calculators. I was a popular "tutor" in Biology, Chemistry, Physics and Math.

But, despite all that I had read, imagined and knew, the chasm between us was great and there was no way to bridge our differences. I mustered all my courage and asked my classmate that I tutored, to our prom; he politely declined. I attended the prom, dressed in a sari, that my mother thought was most appropriate. After all, that is how one would dress for a fancy Indian "function". My classmates complimented me on my appearance, and then painfully avoided me as I watched them ask one another to dance. I was a foreigner in a foreign land.

The next 20 years saw me navigate through arduous experiences that live on as stories in my mind. I adapted by developing an exterior self that was acceptable in Canadian society. My inner self remained content to peer from within.

Then I met my mentor; a brilliant doctor, teacher, innovator and conscientious leader. Under his tutelage, my exterior shell melted away. He was open to passionate discourse and disagreement, and had a way of transmuting it into an enlightening experience. I grew confident to craft original, deeply thought out ideas, speak my mind, air my ideas and debate their merits. Knowing that my mentor valued my ideas seemed to be reason enough to have them.

As my capacity for creative endeavours increased, and I grew in stature and renown, I felt a strange foreboding. One's intuitive self knows more than the eye can see. There were little tugs here and there, during conversations, during meetings, during exchanges. What was once a sandbox full of unrealised potential now resembled an hourglass; something vital was dying.

I recall attending a meeting where the logic model was first introduced to us. I grasped the concepts quickly and pointed out how the presenter could enhance the model by adding feedback arrows within the structure. 'Where were you when I was writing this up', she asked and my heart swelled with pride. I excitedly looked around the room, only to be met with stony silence. My mentor turned his eyes away and left without speaking when the presentation ended. In ensuing meetings, he subtly overruled me, pointing out that he had more experience with the subject matter. When I submitted hours of work on policy documents, he joked that as chair, he could simply delete my ideas and then proceeded to carry it out.

What was happening? What had I done? Why was I being pushed away? What was my mistake? I racked my brain for answers. I trawled the conversations and recent happenings for clues to what I was discerning.

After attending my presentation of an innovative approach to a large audience, my mentor dryly remarked "They will not remember much of this in a month's time". I felt like I was punched in the stomach, but steeled myself to understand the wisdom he was offering in his feedback, that no matter how useful or innovative, people will not remember or absorb new ideas.

Then without warning, he said, 'When you are trying to climb within an organisation, you have to first know your place. Do you know yours?' I was stunned and left speechless. When threatened or vulnerable, animals are known to back down into a docile position, and submit to the power of another. The human animal is no exception. I heard his message. I had overreached and needed to get back down to the place where I belonged.

I regressed and used behaviours that allowed me to coexist, in the male dominated India of my youth. I stopped critically challenging his ideas, choosing instead to limit my contribution to analysis and flattery. I continued to be cautious and careful about bringing new ideas to groups. The less I contributed, the better everything seemed. My concessions appeared to mollify him.

Tacit oppression in interpersonal interactions can result in the victim believing that she deserves the treatment she is receiving. My childhood conditioning made me vulnerable to such victimisation. I felt deeply wounded and suffered in silence. I must have done something to deserve this fall from grace. Maybe he had tried to help me make something of myself, and had failed. This was his way of informing me that I did not make the grade, and I should accept this truth with grace.

Another tenet of victimisation is the longing for validation and the return to the original status quo. It hurt that he did not comment on my increasing silence; he appeared not to notice it. I was disappearing before his very eyes, and it was not visible to him. How could that be? The very act of "seeing me" and recognising my potential, it seemed, was what released me from my original imprisonment. And now, what was I without his approval? Without being validated as being worthy? Without being heard for what I was expressing?

My ship was tossed amidst the stormy seas of crippling self-doubt.

We exist when mirrored in another and I couldn't see myself anymore. The darkness was blinding as it cut through into my light. I could no longer see my inner world. My lamp flickered and threatened to blow out. I stepped away in a desperate act of self-preservation, all the while questioning whether what I perceived as life, laughter and creation were but figments of my own imagination. I pushed away the world that my mentor had introduced. I pushed away from all that was warm, familiar and comfortable. As I grasped the meaning of the writing on the wall, I slowly stepped down from committees; I distanced myself from my mentor and his work; I even stopped participating in mundane meetings about day-to-day affairs; I created an exit strategy and left the organisation with a large void within me.

Nature, however, tolerates a void but for a short time.

I had long wanted to sing, and felt embarrassed by my relatively low register. I grew up listening to female singers with high and melodic voices, not ones with deep and dark tones. I registered for voice lessons with a remarkable teacher.

Somehow, within a few voice lessons, he grasped the root of my discomfort and spoke about it plainly. "There are many female sopranos to be sure, and you have grown up believing their voice range to be desirable for a woman. This is based on what you were conditioned to believe in India. Your voice range is that of a Contralto; which is rare among female singers. You believe it to be undesirable, and have suppressed your voice, its range and its potential. This is affecting you deeply. I want you to hear this poem; you need to know it". I listened to Marianne Williamson's voice in her message:

"Our deepest fear is not that we are inadequate. Our deepest fear is that we are powerful beyond measure. It is our light, not our darkness that most frightens us. We ask ourselves, who am I to be brilliant, gorgeous, talented, and fabulous?"

"Actually, who are you not to be? You are a child of the universe."

"You're playing small does not serve the world. There is nothing enlightened about shrinking so that other people will not feel insecure around you. We are all meant to shine, as children do. We were born to make manifest the glory of the universe that is within us. It is not just in some of us; it is in everyone and as we let our own light shine, we unconsciously give others permission to do the same. As we are liberated from our own fear, our presence automatically liberates others."

These powerful words have since guided my light.

I thank my first mentor for the gift of the sugar-coated bitter pill; as its bitterness became evident, it caused me great pain and consternation. It caused my shipwreck. And as I experienced isolation while cast aside, I felt it all the more acutely, having known the warmth and comfort of togetherness. But that voyage freed me from the imprisonment of ego gratification. My mentor, however, remains a prisoner. His inability to rise above the fear of losing power when blinded by the light of another is now evident to me.

My next mentor taught me that true power lies within each of us. We are given many chances to choose it with free will: it is always within our grasp. When we align our ego and efforts with our inner pilot light, we are rewarded with insight, wisdom, compassion, empathy, love and peace. We can see each other as we truly are and seek to guide, coach, and uplift one another with our life force.

And you, dear reader, have you ever been drawn out of your shell by the sweetness of a sugar-coated pill; by the promise of a fairy tale ending; by the comfort of being bubble wrapped?

As you step outside the shadow cast by your ego, your light shines brighter. It brings light to paths that were previously invisible.

Welcome to the life of voyage. Our ships are built to sail, and sail each one will. We will face storms, wreck over shoals and be stranded. In our darkest hours, our light still shines, leading others to our aid and leading us to others. Thus, we break through the bubble wrap that insulates us from essential elements of human relationships—both sweet and bitter.

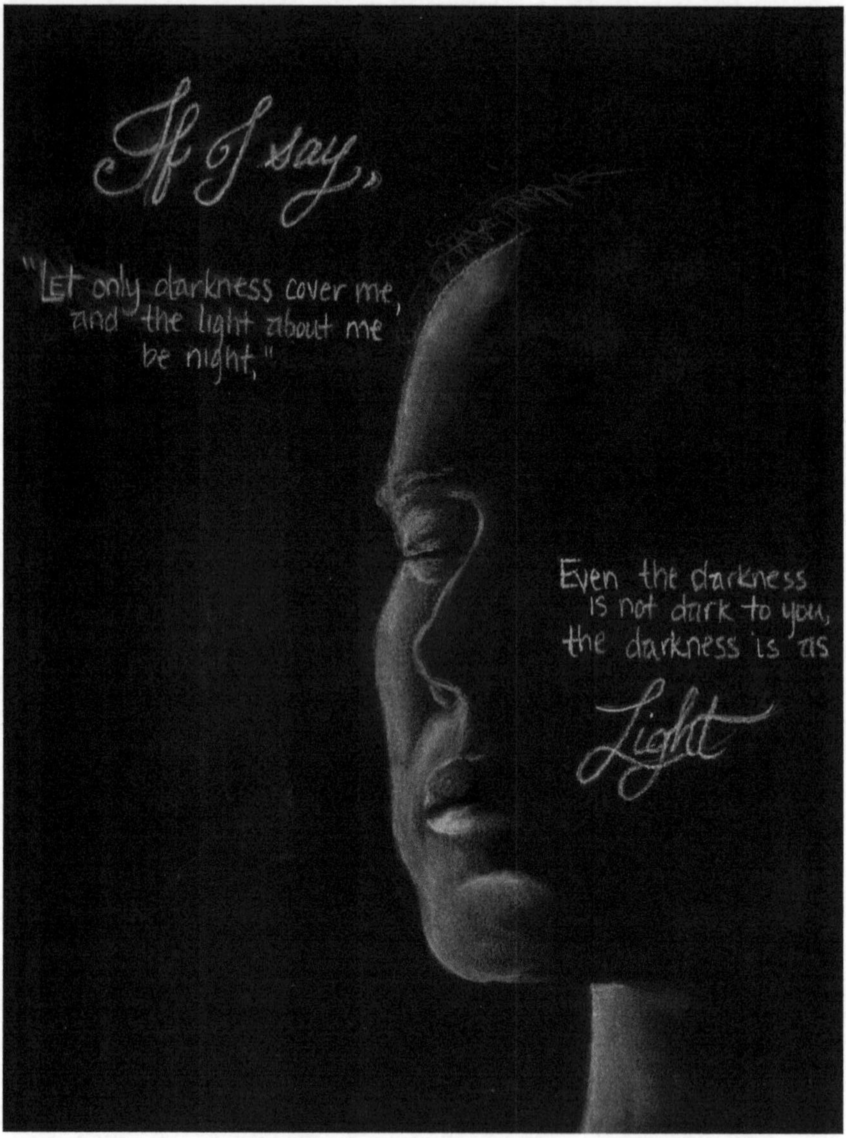
If I say,
"Let only darkness cover me, and the light about me be night,"
Even the darkness is not dark to you, the darkness is as
Light

"I'm Not Sure How to Tell You This..."

David B. Seaburn

They are talking to each other in hushed tones about daily things. Her black hair is in disarray and her arms, resting on the top sheet of her hospital bed, are gaunt, her skin like onion paper. Yet she smiles as we enter, and I can see youth in her darkened eyes. Her husband turns in his chair, his face drawn and weary, and his grin polite. Their eleven-year-old son is in school. As a behavioral health faculty, I am here to support a family medicine resident who is about to give unwelcome news for the first time.

The resident had come to my office a day earlier to tell me she had a young mother in the hospital who had been in cancer treatment for a considerable period of time. The resident had just learned from the patient's oncologist that there was nothing more to be done, that the cancer was now sweeping through her body, relentless. The resident, having developed a close relationship with the family, wanted to be the bearer of this news. But she was unsure of what to do, so she consulted with me.

We talked about some basic guidelines for talking with patients about what most would consider bad news, a kind of protocol, recognizing that it was often done poorly, that the anxiety of the provider could easily get in the way, that any hurriedness might leave the patient and loved ones befuddled and frustrated. It would be useful to start by asking the patient and her husband how they thought things were going and what their hopes for the future were. This would give the resident a baseline upon which to build. Using jargon-free lay language would be critical to insure clarity. Pausing so the patient has time to digest information and formulate questions would be crucial. Repeating the information a second time, and perhaps a third, would help the patient and her husband absorb what the resident was telling them. Listening for feelings would be vital, too. Each of these steps would help a difficult situation go more smoothly.

At the end our conversation, the resident still looked wary. I offered to go to the hospital with her for support or guidance, if needed. And so it was that we found ourselves together with the patient and husband in the drab green confines of her hospital room.

After a brief greeting and introduction, the resident begins: "I have some news I want to share with you. The treatments are no longer effective. I'm afraid nothing more can be done. When you die, it will be from this cancer." At first, the patient, her eyes glancing elsewhere, ignores what she has been told while her husband sits in stunned silence. Then, the patient melts into tears and asks the resident to tell her again, which she does. The patient and her husband hold each other for a long time, silent; then their hands fold over their faces as they think of their son. They ask again—"What are you telling us?"—followed by tears, more questions, confusion, changes in subject to relieve the enveloping despair, silence again. Their doctor stays with them throughout, holds their hands, is quiet, acknowledges what she doesn't know, sheds tears. Despite the necessity of professional boundaries between physicians and their patients, she is now a part of them and they are a part of her.

We came to the hospital with a map, but learned quickly that it matched the territory in only a general way. There wasn't an apt protocol for handling the emotions evoked by news that one's life was ending soon and that one's husband and young son would be left behind. Nothing could sweep away the fog that was ebbing; nothing could illuminate the cavernous darkness that lay ahead. The best that the resident physician could do was enter the darkness with them, settle there for a time, embrace them, and seek a way forward even when a pathway did not readily present itself.

I could not help but think of Psalm 139 from the Old Testament which says the strangest of things: "If I say, 'Let only darkness cover me, and the light about me be night,' even the darkness is not dark to you, the darkness is as light…" For years, I thought the writer was talking about the commonplace image of light shining in darkness. But this experience and others helped me understand it differently. Sometimes darkness itself is the only light afforded us. It is inescapable; something we all face.

And when we enter there, we see that all we can do is hold onto whoever is willing to go there with us. The experience of holding on or being held is sacred, even when the light it casts may seem invisible. It is, nevertheless, enough to make it through. As this young physician walked with them into a darkened future, she learned that when there is no cure, and the light seems extinguished, the simple yet courageous act of being there can be healing.

Beyond Functional Gait

John Spangler

I ran into Chip at the gym today. He had been my mentor for two decades.

He is about 10 years my elder. I hadn't seen him in a few years, and he looked great. Really, the best I have seen him in a long, long while.

We chatted about old times when he amazed me with his clinical acumen and his skills I wished I could master. He had such supple confidence and efficiency.

He attended every morning report and noon conference asking insightful questions as a way of teaching residents and medical students. When I gave talks, there was no question he could not answer. Yet he held off answering to allow learners to learn. He would only answer if there were no learned-enough learners. His answers were neither showboats nor one word.

He taught as he answered, as natural as sunshine.

While precepting residents in clinic, he knew the diagnosis of the most perplexing cases. I'd curbside him frequently. When I was an intern, he was my favorite attending; you knew your day was going to be efficient with him as boss.

His patients adored him. He had many geriatric patients, a qualification-certified field he loved. He got to know his elders deeply, and they trusted him implicitly. They received every vaccine, mammogram, and colonoscopy on time. They were up to date on all diabetes and hypertension guidelines.

He was skilled with his hands, too. In the military, he learned how to do simple vasectomies, sigmoidoscopies, colonoscopies—plus the usual dark-spot punches and elliptical biopsies of more ominous lesions.

Often theatrical, he sang beautifully at church, in plays and at various residency events.

He was a family role model too, an engaged dad and husband. I would see him and Joan, his wife, walking in the neighborhood, holding hands.

Probably walking home from their favorite frozen yogurt shop 4 blocks away.

We all noticed their joyful love.

Their love remains, still as devoted to each other and to their cabin in the Pocono Mountains as he formerly was to golf and geriatrics. Indeed, they both still brim with hope that is incongruous with what befell him.

> Two decades my mentor, one decade my senior, a half decade post-stroke—in his wake, I realize I am still becoming a learned learner.

His wooded landscaped lot grew out of his zest for life. Its cool-breezed solace still shades flowers of reds and yellows and hosts bluebirds colored sunset and sky.

But life darkly punched him down half a dozen years ago. Chip became uncharacteristically blue. But wouldn't you? After such a vital love of life? Of singing, acting, and of golf?

One night Chip awoke with a headache. With Joan and abundant caution, he hastened to the hospital. After a benign ED work-up—and feeling better—they repaired back home.

That morning, he seemed okay. He and a second year resident visited patients in the nursing home as part of her geriatrics rotation. The way I heard it, he suddenly appeared stricken, syncopal, and fell to the floor insensible—like a punch, like a stroke.

With immediate transport to our hospital, he had emergent neurovascular surgery, a prolonged stay in the neurosurgical ICU, and transfer to a physical rehabilitation facility. This spirited, brilliant, singer-scholar—now silenced on his vocal side and weakened on his right.

We were also struck dumb. Who will so elegantly teach the first year students' Doctor Patient Relationship course? Who will model geriatrics to our residents? Sing at resident graduations? Staff morning report so faithfully?

Who will so adroitly craft board questions for national medical students as a National Board Examiner?

What we all really wanted to know was how someone so vital just vanishes.

I saw him once coming to clinic for a checkup. I reached out my right hand to shake his; he grasped my hand with his left. I felt so completely gauche neglecting his new right-sided reality and his halting speech. I obtusely asked how he was doing.

"It's. In. My. Mind. Thoughts," he replied.

Long pause.

"In. Brain."

The next I heard from him was a form letter, with a personal handwritten note at the bottom, advocating for cognitive rehabilitation, something I knew nothing about. His letter explained that there is little awareness among physicians of cognitive rehab's existence. There is even less awareness about its efficacy in getting patients post-stroke closer to their baseline intellectual capabilities.

I later learned Chip testified before Congress advocating for cognitive rehab funding.

And then today, there he was in the lobby of the gym.

I reached out my left hand this time, shook his left hand, and embraced him in a man hug.

"Chip, it's so wonderful to see you!"

"It's great to see you too, John. It's been a while."

I was astonished! Chip was nearly fluent. He was confident, more muscular, his friendliness brightly on display again.

"Chip, we miss you. I remember how you encouraged me as an intern, supported my early career with such apt advice."

He smiled as he shook his head as if to say, modestly, no, not me.

"Honestly, Chip! You were one of our most brilliant clinicians—and such a good friend to boot! You were nationally recognized in medical education. You sang. You excelled in sports. You loved to play golf. You acted in the Little Theater."

I paused to check his reaction.

"Remember the song you composed about Katie and Alice? Chief residents 15 years ago? Capable, bright residents, so compassionate? You sang that song at their graduation. Few eyes were dry."

"Come on, John. I simply lived what I loved," he said evenly.

"If that's the case, you loved a lot and you lived a lot. You taught a lot. We all loved and still love you—a lot!"

He smiled as we gently embraced again, and, turning, he headed to the locker room, about 20 feet away.

He reached the locker room door in 5 seconds. I counted, as if assessing his gait. He displayed no imbalance or deviation in his walk width. His stride was smooth with a regular cadence.

As he turned his head and waved goodbye to me, his speed did not slow down.

Just as his life has not slowed down.

His stroke simply turned his head. With that turn, he picked himself off the nursing home floor and pivoted in a new direction.

Two decades my mentor, one decade my senior, a half decade post-stroke—in his wake, I realize I am still becoming a learned learner.

And his new, redirected gait is beyond functional.

It is pioneering.

* * *

Acknowledgements I would like to thank Chip and Joan for their willingness to allow publication of this essay.

Knee Touch Moments

Andrew S. Valeras

"I am not sure that it makes a difference, but I like to believe it does," Dr. George Devito taught me 9 years ago. I was a family medicine intern who had just completed an overwhelming well-child check with a rambunctious 4 year old. This visit was similar in the level of chaos to many well-child checks that we had done together that month as part of my Outpatient Pediatrics Rotation. Four weeks—a mere 20 days—to prepare me for everything there was to know about caring for humans less than 18 years of age.

Many were too young to speak. Many were teenagers that would not speak, choosing to sit coolly with an aphasia-stricken apathy for adults. At the time, I did not have kids of my own to experiment with and learn on, so Dr. Devito was all I had to illuminate the wonders of this complicated and terrifying cohort of my future career in Family Medicine. The ever-resilient, yet unmistakably fragile, developing child is a paradox no medical training can prepare one to fully understand. Understanding and sensing are very different things, however.

Dr. Devito, known to all as Skip, cared for children and adolescents for 38 years as a practicing pediatrician, and cared for new Family Medicine Residents, like myself, for almost as long. His salt and pepper beard was seemingly grown as something young patients could reach for and occupy their gaze, as they looked up from the exam table.

Skip's niche was pediatric behavioral concerns. He addressed the concerns of the patient, those of the parents, and those of the schoolteachers. At the residency, he also addressed the needs of the physicians-in-training that did not know what to do next, other than to "call Skip." He guided residents in understanding the nuances of how neonates, infants, and young children express their medical and emotional needs and in ensuring that the parents could interpret and translate the language of cries, grunts, soft heads banging against hard floors, or pants soiled as an act of defiance.

Through his years of experience, Skip became the Rosetta Stone of pediatric care, a masterful decoder that all family physicians would strive for in order to aptly treat this population. This alone would have been sufficient in the technical delivery of effective pediatric care. For those training in healthcare in the modern electronic era, success has come to mean a completed note, in a timely fashion, with all the buttons clicked for the quality metrics of the month. Dr. Devito was more interested in the narrative however—the narrative told by the patient, parents, and caregivers; the narrative observed and interpreted by the clinician; and most importantly, the narrative yet to be told. He was a master of embracing the future narrative, with all the potential and possibility embodied in a child's life.

> Though many would assume predestination, with the gentlest of gestures, Skip sought to influence the trajectory with hope.

The context of a child's life often dictates the narrative told. The unfolding of a story of poverty, lack of education, single parenting sometimes matched the narrative observed in the room—strain between mother and child, imbalance between parenting and working, a father with a pained expression considering how to feed the family the recommended healthy food to prevent further worsening of obesity. But sometimes the story told defies the narrative observed—a family with all odds stacked against them thriving in the chaos, holding onto hope and parenting poise.

Skip took in these narratives and focused on the future one. Though many would assume predestination, with the gentlest of gestures, Skip sought to influence the trajectory with hope.

Over his career, Skip learned when a connection was needed, to reach out. Skip would make a physical connection, a hand gently placed on the knee, not as the act, but as the prelude. Once he had the parent's attention amidst the exam room chaos, eye contact made with 2 learned and soulful eyes above a graying beard, he would deliver a simple yet reverberating message:

"You are doing a great job as a parent. Your child is lucky to have you as a parent." Then Skip would release the visit back to the chaos, close out the encounter, and move on to the next patient, the next resident, the next narrative, over and over for 38 years.

When I became an attending, I was also adapting to my role as a father to 3 young children. The trials of sleepless nights, hard parenting decisions, and the flood of doubts and concerns that I was somehow ruining the future narrative of young souls constantly weighed on me. I always had Skip to reassure me though: "You're doing just fine. They are lucky to have you and Aimee as their parents." I incorporated his message into my own practice as well.

Over time, I have learned the skill of how to capture the fleeting attention of a sleep-deprived parent lost in worry, to connect and say the words, "You are doing a great job as a parent. Look how well your son is growing. You did that. He is so lucky to have you." The words might change slightly, but the message is always the same: a gesture of hope that a future narrative would be a little bit more promising and a little easier to see. I tried to pass on Skip's habit of whispering through time, nudging a future in which a child was yelled at once less, was allowed to be a child a little longer, was encouraged to succeed. I aimed to foretell a future in which parents did not doubt their child or themselves, even when everyone's prediction was failure.

I thought I was doing this for the parent whose knee my hand rested upon, but I realized over time it was really for me. It gives me the semblance of meaning, that we, as physicians, can make a difference in the narratives of our patients. Seeing children with boundless opportunity makes it even harder to take in the harsh realities of a world in which they are often powerless. I've held onto this practice not knowing if it has an impact; I lacked the faith Skip carried within him that this mattered.

My doubts, however, diminished when a note arrived. It was a plain handwritten scrawl on a white sheet of paper torn in half inside an envelope with only my professional name on front. It read:

"Thank you. My son's well-child visit with you was the first time I heard, in my whole life, that I was doing a good job as a mom. I have been doubting my parenting for years, to the point of crying myself to sleep. Being a mom is the hardest thing I have done, and everyone tells me to do it better. That day was the first day I was told I'm doing ok, and it made all the difference."

I read the note several times to soak it all in. Once I had saturated myself in the words, I ran across the hallway, note held high to catch the light, to Skip's office. He was packing the multitude of pediatric books from which he taught, clearing away all the technical aspects of his craft into cardboard boxes for a well-deserved retirement from clinical practice. I exclaimed, "Skip, it works! Knee touch moments matter. Here is the proof!"

As I read the note out loud, Skip smiled and touched me gently on the shoulder, "You are doing a really great job as a doctor, Andy." And it made all the difference.

Mentoring Connections:
Helping Trainees Give the Best of Themselves

Kathryn Fraser and Claudia Allen

Mentoring: Above and Below the Surface

"The delicate balance of mentoring someone is not creating them in your own image, but giving them the opportunity to create themselves."

Stephen Spielberg

No one really knows what is expected of them when they are asked to be a mentor. We had the pleasure of being involved in the Behavioral Science/Family Systems' Education Fellowship (BFEF), a mentoring project for early career Behavioral Science Faculty (BSF) in Family Medicine Residency education. Kathryn was a small-group Co-Mentor and then was the "Meta-Mentor" who guided Claudia and the other Small-Group Co-Mentors. Our task was to help new faculty hone their teaching skills and get clarity on their roles. This project created an unforgettable journey, and brought these mentors rewards that seemed even greater than what the mentees received at times.

Kathryn's Story

Connecting with mentees in the BFEF is really about helping them become knowledgeable in a field that is secondary to their training as mental health providers, i.e., Family Medicine. My co-mentor and I felt privileged to hear about the challenges and the struggles of our fellows. We mostly started out talking about what was lacking in everyone's curriculum and how to use the latest, jazziest teaching techniques.

I distinctly recall the moment when one of our mentees started to go in a direction that was obviously painful. We could all see a change in facial expression, somewhere between loss and utter defeat. Clearly, they questioned their abilities based on how their learners were responding to them. I remember my co-mentor encouraged the person to "stick with it" as this emotion bubbled up. This moment was life altering for me because we changed the dynamic in our group and saw the potential for true growth and deep change. We could have simply continued to focus on the task and avoid the deeper process that we could use to effect change, but we didn't. Here was an opportunity to help a peer who, on the surface, appeared to "have everything" but was in great need. As a group, we trusted each other and were willing to take the risk of exposing more intense emotions so that we could all grow...together.

> Some of our richest mentor–mentee conversations involved helping each other find the courage to step up when we had something valuable to offer, and the wisdom to ask for help rather than carry the load alone.

The term "Small Group" gave us a sense of belonging and became a great theme for the goal of creating a supportive community. My identity as a "Small Group Mentor" (SGM) began to form and the specialness of that designation was not lost on me. In many ways, our group dynamic felt like "peer mentoring" because it was evident that we were all in the same boat struggling with our identities, though my co-mentor and I were further along in our journeys. We developed wonderful social relationships, perhaps born of this shared mutual pain. There was an ease among the six of us. We alternated between talking about the best parts of our lives and then switching the conversation to helping each other figure out how to navigate tricky professional situations. In trying to figure out what my mentees needed, I found my most important instrument was my authentic self. I didn't feel I was teaching them much about completing tasks per se, but more about connecting with who they really were—what was important to them, their values and beliefs.

The term "Meta Mentor," a role I assumed two years later, also seemed to be deliberately chosen. I was to "mentor the mentors," not "lead" or "supervise" them. This required that same deliberate listening, joining, empathizing, and daring to risk revealing my own challenges. I would have three calls with the SGMs during the year to check in, learn about each fellow's progress, and offer support in any way I could. Along the way, I realized that my unique ability to be very "relational," as the BFEF Director told me, was key to my role. I can accept a wide variety of personalities, be genuinely empathetic and supportive, confront when necessary, and push others to their growing edges. It turns out that teaching others to do that also seemed to come naturally. Oddly enough, I feel that many of my capabilities with meta mentoring stemmed from my own early career experiences which were fraught with insecurity, shame, self-doubt, and self-criticism. How far I had come since then!

Claudia's work as a mentor stood out for me in that she brought a sense of structure and fluidity to her mentoring style. She took her job seriously in terms of providing guidance, but also learned quickly that she would not have all the answers. Sometimes, the mentor's role is to help the mentee contain their stress of not knowing, while remaining productive and high functioning. She became a model for them to gracefully move in and out of those spaces of confidence and skill to the rougher territory of the "incomplete knowledge base"—moments that tug at your self-image.

Claudia's Story

My role in the fellowship has been twofold: as both an SGM to 2 sets of fellows and simultaneously as a mentee to Kathryn in her role as Meta Mentor. Parallel process comes into play, and in this case in a very positive way. Mentoring is a delicate dance of providing some guidance and inspiration, but not controlling one's mentees. From "the top down," Kathryn has skillfully modeled that dance, communicating to all her SGMs that she trusts their skills and instincts, yet is available for consultation and support. We absorbed this attitude, and it made us more inclined to take that approach with our own mentees. This allowed our conference calls with our fellows to go deeper than the required research projects. We discussed sensitive professional issues such as how to self-advocate for adequate pay, how to talk about race, how best to navigate departmental politics, and how to help our colleagues grieve tragic deaths while grieving ourselves. As SGMs, my co-mentor and I also delved into personal matters such as deaths in our own families, our own feelings of burnout, and our struggles balancing work and family.

The mentees each came from a unique environment, so the conversations varied far and wide. The mentees' toughest professional struggles often seemed to involve situations where they found themselves supporting learners, colleagues, or whole departments through some kind of emotional crisis. Some examples of this included death of a patient or colleague, fallout from unprofessional behavior, or toxic interpersonal conflict. Helping their departments weather these crises was not specifically in the mentees' job descriptions, and there certainly wasn't a roadmap, but they often found themselves in a unique position to offer something that perhaps no one else could, even if they were unsure if it was their "place" to do that.

Some of our richest mentor–mentee conversations involved helping each other find the courage to step up when we had something valuable to offer, and the wisdom to ask for help rather than carry the load alone. One thing that has surprised me is how useful it is to share a current struggle of my own and think about it aloud with my mentees—not just to share "the answers." This thinking out loud as a group seemed to be where we got our best work done, and providing a space for that has been one of my most productive approaches. In observing Kathryn's mentoring of the SGMs, I absorbed permission to be myself as a mentor, to offer my mentees my best listening ear, my experience, and my interest in them, rather than a list of "how to's." Don't get me wrong, "how to" advice does get sprinkled in, but I have learned as many tips and tricks from my mentees as I have taught them. What my mentees seemed to crave was a space to talk about how they and their behavioral skills fit in their medical programs.

Developing a Shared Vision

This phrase represents a parallel process that happened between us (Kathryn and Claudia) as Meta Mentor and Small-Group Mentor, and also happened with each one of us and our mentee groups. Good listening, giving direction, empathizing, and leading by example took us to a place where a shared vision could develop. Mentors in the behavioral sciences are uniquely positioned to understand multiple layers of dynamics in the mentor–mentee relationship. Mentors walk a fine line with the ethics of professional boundaries that require us to get close but not too close and be directive but not too directive. Ultimately, the mentees must stand on their own, and also deal with all types of personalities. The strong mentor–mentee relationship prepares them for this, and simultaneously helps them demand the best of people around them. Mentoring is truly about helping someone learn to strive for the highest aspirations of their professional self. We can all walk away from those types of relationships with dignity, improved self-confidence, and hopefully a desire to keep aspiring for our best selves.

Strong Mentors: May We Know Them. May We Be Them

Laura Sudano and Florencia Lebensohn-Chialvo

Laura Sudano

I was 19 years old and just completed my first year in collegiate volleyball. A year earlier, my coach told me that after one year of commitment to the team, I would be eligible for a scholarship.

I walked across campus rehearsing how to approach such a conversation.

I would like to talk with you about the opportunity for a scholarship. No, too upfront, I thought. I should anchor the conversation, so they aren't blindsided.

You mentioned that I would be eligible for a scholarship around this time last year. Can we talk about this? Maybe, but still this seems awkward. Should I be the one to bring this up?

I made my way down the steps and to the basement of the prehistoric athletic building; the type of structure where the rubber-matted flooring hasn't been changed for over 40 years and still has the sweat of the hundreds of athletes in its pores. The cold, white-painted cinder block walls offered no inspiration or comfort. *I hate this walk.* The office was down three corridors—2 long and 1 short—where you would find the man in the iron mask.

My feet finally reached the office door. I entered, carefully observing what their mood was that day almost as a way to predict the outcome of the conversation. I had only asked my parents for money up until this point. Unlike my parents, this is a person who has the capability of granting me permission to play in games, can sit me out during practice, demand that I run extra during weights or practice, and moreover, can deny my stability that would be important for me at this stage of my life.

I don't know exactly what I said, but it was a mishmash of the least awkward openings developed during my mental gymnastics on the way to their office. Although those details are fuzzy, I am clear about the response: "You have a million-dollar contract with Nike. I don't know why you're asking me this."

The nanosecond, which takes five seconds to explain, internal conversation happened.

I do? I don't understand. This was a mistake coming to talk about this with them. Wait. Are they talking about me, the team, or

> We step up and back, all the while supporting each other in our career endeavors.

school? It's not me. Nike gave the school a million dollars? That is a lot of money. How do they come to that number? Is that what it costs to operate a Division I athletics program? Did my partner know that Nike gave a million dollars in gear to athletics? Is this a no? What do I say? Say something.

Focus.

I was in uncharted territory without a map. And in retrospect, I think they too were empty handed to walk through this unknown land with me. Or, at the very least, they were familiar with these types of conversations and wanted to shut it down quickly.

Other words were exchanged, such as an explanation about how the conference player of the year at a different school was a senior who didn't have a scholarship. *Should I just be grateful to be on the team? That I have a million-dollar contract with Nike? That there are people who are deserving of opportunities and aren't awarded, accordingly?*

Little did I know that I would continue to encounter this situation with others in the professional world after my collegiate experience. The experiences weren't in the form of someone telling me that I have a million-dollar contract with Nike. It looked more like buying the academia bill of goods.

That is, I was told that the academic work would be a collaboration. I would go forward and mail out recruitment letters, call participants to do interventions, collect data, write a grant, set up the electronic health record system to capture data, and train the behavioral health workforce. But at the end, the senior faculty published a manuscript and/or presented at national organizations unbeknownst to me.

Gratefully, I've also had positive relationships with mentors in which I had an opportunity to lay the groundwork and they provided the scaffolding. I appreciate the opportunity that these individuals presented to co-write manuscripts and co-present findings at national conferences.

It is easier to reflect on these times after years have passed. From this, I've learned that honesty and transparency are characteristics I value. I am conscientious of it in my relationship to mentees and mentors. This quality has been most notable in mentor relationships where I seek guidance, and their wisdom is reflected in the way in which they have handled their career. And more importantly, how they have navigated relationships with others—leadership, peers, students, and early career professionals.

* * *

Florencia Lebensohn-Chialvo

My first year as an assistant professor went surprisingly well. By all indications, I was settling into my teaching and supervision and handling my service responsibilities well. I felt good about the collegial relationships I had forged and I still had time and energy left over at the end of the day for my husband and children.

Hey, this whole being an academic thing isn't as hard as I thought it would be...

I was in no way prepared for the roller coaster ride that awaited me. Over the next year, I encountered situations with students, colleagues, and in my home life that chipped away at the confidence I had built up and I started doubting whether I was cut out for the job.

But, I don't want to exaggerate things. By and large, I had wonderful interactions with students. They were curious, engaged, and eager to learn. There were a select few, however, who challenged me in all the wrong ways. They were constantly dissatisfied with how I presented material in class or how I answered their questions about clinical dilemmas. In some ways I could empathize with these students—they needed to know what the "right" answer was to all potential scenarios, which wasn't something I could necessarily provide. This resulted in frustrated office hour visits and less than perfect course evaluations.

It wasn't long before I started questioning my teaching methods and falling into the same trap as these students, asking myself, *"Am I doing this right?"* I had also become preoccupied with how students were interacting with the other senior faculty in my program. *Wow, do they make similar demands of the others? Do they think they can push me around because I'm the most junior faculty member?* And probably most disturbing, I started noticing how these distractions were coming home with me. Way too often, I would be at the dinner table with my children, still replaying a conversation with a student in my head or second guessing an email I had sent to a colleague. *This is not good...Why can't I turn it off?*

As that academic year was coming to a close, it was time for my annual evaluation meeting with my department chair, who over those 2 years had become an important mentor to me. When I first joined the department, I had been *very* intimidated by her. She was a nationally renowned scholar, a highly regarded member of our professional community, and a skilled administrator. Yet, I quickly realized that one of her greatest skills was engaging me in conversation and creating a space for authentic and non-judgmental reflection. She also had a way of conveying her genuine desire to see everyone succeed–however members of her faculty defined success.

After we had gone over all the required sections, I noticed my heart rate accelerate and my ability to focus start to wean, as tends to happen when I know I'm about to venture into the uncomfortable. *If I don't talk about it now, it's going to continue to eat at me.*

"I'm just not sure students respect me all that much. They don't treat me the same way as they do the others...or maybe they do and I'm being overly sensitive...I don't know what I'm doing wrong...if I'm doing something wrong..." I trailed off, not sure what I wanted to say or what I felt comfortable putting words to.

"I can see that this is really impacting you and I think I know what you mean but why don't you explain it to me a bit more."

What followed was a lot of me working up the courage to be fully honest with myself, trusting that doing so wouldn't erode the confidence she had in my abilities. *Why didn't I do this sooner!* I was allowed to share freely, never feeling rushed or that words were being put in my mouth. She emphasized and normalized my experience while gently encouraging me to focus on what I had control over to change my circumstances for the better.

I'd like to say there was some major epiphany or decision that came out of the discussion—but there wasn't. It did, however, lead me to engage in more critical conversations with myself and others about what sort of educator, supervisor, mentor, working wife, and mother I wanted to be.

Who do I feel equipped to mentor? Who am I interested in mentoring and why? What parts of myself do I feel comfortable sharing with mentees? What parts of myself do I want to keep for myself? For my family and loved ones? Who do I want to emulate? Or do I forge my own path?

And while I am still very much just getting started on this journey, I have come to appreciate and value a couple of things; if I operate from my values and remain true to myself, I will reach the mentees who most need my version of mentorship and those that don't will likely find their right match somewhere else—and that's just plain OK.

* * *

We are mindful of our differences, our strengths, and shared experiences. We step up and back, all the while supporting each other in our career endeavors. These experiences that we have—be they with disingenuous or compassionate mentors —shape us. They inform who we seek out, who we strive to be, and who we eventually become.

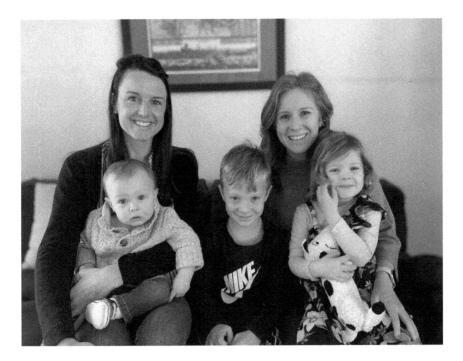

An Unlikely Path to Meaning and Mentorship

Michael M. Talamantes and John Scheid

John: It was two weeks before my wedding, and something felt off. Really off. How could that be possible? I was about to marry my best friend of 15 years. Menus were set, the forecast was clear, and we found the perfect streamside meadow at the foot of our favorite mountain to share with the most important people in our lives. In fact, we managed to infuse meaning and nostalgia into virtually every aspect of the day. We spent the previous year propagating table centerpieces from our own plants, the place card design integrated a concert ticket stub from the night we met, and the ceremony site included a sculpture of my late father's favorite bird to honor him during the ceremony. It was us.

Then, it hit me. Meghan and I had so much meaningful history together. We literally spent half our lives making memories before even getting married. Everyone in attendance knew the saga of our relationship, but we only met our officiant a scant few months prior. He was friendly enough, but he didn't know us. I felt as though we needed an officiant who was a close friend but could also offer direction, guidance, and experience. That's when I sent Michael a message he never could have predicted when he accepted me as an intern five years prior: "How long do you think it would take to get a license to marry someone in CO? Just food for thought."

Michael: After speaking to 25 other students that afternoon, John was the last student whom I spoke with at the internship recruitment fair. He had a confidence about him along with maturity that I had not noticed with the other students. He interviewed with me and spent some time with me during interdisciplinary rounds. We had a good camaraderie from the start. He was relaxed and had good questions. I thought that his laid back attitude might be a good contrast to my more uptight approach. John eventually accepted his graduate MSW internship at the transplant clinic with me and he appeared like any of the prior 20 MSW students that I had supervised…young, enthusiastic, and ambitious. John would begin in the fall.

John: 2013 marked a pivotal state of my life. At the time, I heavily confided in my dad who was a psychologist. We enjoyed discussing clinical cases and reviewing my documentation. I sought his advice and direction regarding various aspects of graduate school. I embraced dad's counsel to pursue clinical training in an academic hospital setting. Unbeknownst to me, this would be one of his final gifts of advice, as dad passed away unexpectedly just prior to my internship.

My world changed in an instant. I was packing my car to visit my parents before leaving the country to work in New Zealand for the summer. I didn't have my phone with me, and Meghan rushed outside with a perplexed look of concern to tell me that she

While I had my reservations about his emotional well-being, I could not deny him this opportunity. In hindsight, I was also concerned about my own well-being. You see, I also lost my dad under eerily similar circumstances.

had repeated missed calls from my mom. She placed the phone in my hands, almost to ensure that I relieved her from its weight. I immediately responded to mom's distress signals, and her first words were, "He's gone. John…I'm so sorry. Your dad is gone." I collapsed in a pile of defeat, and Meghan met me at the ground to offer an empathetic embrace. She knew. Through tears and a broken voice that wasn't my own, I asked mom what happened and if she was okay. "It was a heart attack," she responded, "he's gone." I was supposed to see him the very next day.

Michael: I found out about John's father's death from my daughter, who worked with Meghan. It saddened me deeply to hear this news and I was also very concerned as to whether this would be the right internship for John. I wanted to meet with John to discuss this with him.

John: Two qualities intrigued me about Michael: his sensitive yet straightforward demeanor paired with a component of solemnity that exuded seriousness. Several weeks before my internship began, I received a kind-hearted email from him that broke from the mold of formality he applied when relaying logistics and informative content. I knew he heard the news of my dad's passing through his daughter. His email still took me by surprise:

Hello John,

My daughter Sarah told me (as Meghan had told her) about your father. I am so sorry to hear that. I remember talking about him with you on at least 2 different occasions and know how special he was to you. I do not know exactly when it happened, but it must have been shortly before you left. Know that I have been thinking about you and your family at this time. I believe that you were planning on going home at the end of August? I hope you are still planning to go to be with your family. I hope we can talk about this more in September. If I can be of any help, please let me know.

Take care John and I look forward to seeing you in a few weeks.

Michael

In hindsight, this foreshadowed what I would come to learn about Michael—his passion, gravity, experience, and frankness would prove integral in the conception of a deeply meaningful relationship.

Michael: When John and I met prior to the commencement of the internship, I was concerned that John's significant loss was too fresh and I recommended that he consider finding another internship, one that did not involve grief and loss as frequently as we dealt with on the transplant team. With tears in his eyes, he said, "My dad recommended that I do this internship at a teaching institution. I still would like to do my internship here and I think I can do it."

While I had my reservations about his emotional well-being, I could not deny him this opportunity. In hindsight, I was also concerned about my own well-being. You see, I also lost my dad under eerily similar circumstances. Perhaps I knew that if John worked with me, that I would have to deal with my own unresolved grief issues regarding my own father's death in 1985 when I was 21 years old. In spite of this, I agreed that John would start his internship with me in September.

The first few weeks of the internship were fairly typical. John quickly became oriented to the role while occasionally being overwhelmed by the medical terminology, the system, and the team's expectations of the social worker. As John became more autonomous and confident in his understanding of how to help patients and families deal with loss, the death of his father and ability to cope with his strong emotions loomed large during our weekly supervision time. While our supervision time certainly focused on his professional growth and his acquisition of the social work competencies, John needed space to discuss the death of his father and how this impacted his role as a social worker. Since John's dad was a psychologist, it often felt like a natural discussion about how John was dealing with his own grief.

When my own dad died, I was too young and immature to process my feelings. Or perhaps I never had the right person in my life to help me facilitate this process. I did the only thing I felt I could do which was to move on, take care of my widowed mother, and proceed with my education, career, and relationships. While there was now a significant void in my life, I was great about compartmentalizing those feelings, for better or worse.

John: Initially, our supervision was education-oriented and objective, but Michael did share that he also lost his father at a young age. In an attempt to separate my personal life from my professional life, I appreciated his self-disclosure but did not overtly welcome discussion surrounding my own loss at that time. I took the summer to be with my mom and process my dad's passing. I was intentional about my grief and felt ready to move forward.

This is when Michael revealed his true colors. He knew better. Within a month of our mentor–mentee relationship, he forged a conversation about my dad by relating it to the meaningful and privileged work of supporting individuals facing life-threatening diagnoses. This was a defining moment in our relationship. Nobody inquired as directly about my dad as Michael did in that conversation. Despite my best efforts to stifle my emotions, tears swelled, and I broke down in front of a man I hardly knew. When I raised my head from my hands, I was shocked to see that Michael was crying as well.

As much as I attempted to conceal my emotions, Michael possessed a natural and genuine approach to supervision. I will never forget his emotional response to me breaking down about my dad. I knew at that instant that I had much more in common with my mentor than I initially thought.

Michael: I don't think it was easy for John. We would start out discussing clinical cases, assessments and interventions, and team dynamics but almost always ended up talking about our dads. We frequently lost track of time. John discussed aspects of his relationship with his father that were most memorable for him. These memories often revolved around their time together in the Northwoods of Wisconsin, of fishing and of loons and of deep conversations they shared about John's future. These were often emotional conversations for both of us. As John became more vulnerable during our discussions, somehow, this helped me begin to better understand my own feelings and share some of these with John that had been buried for over 30 years. John was a good listener and open to my recol-lections of my own distant memories. We rarely looked at our watches and would often leave the hospital late. I always looked forward to our conversations.

John: As our mentor–mentee relationship progressed, Michael and I realized similarities and challenged one another's differences in mostly respectable fash-ions. When Michael accepted a full-time teaching position at the University of Denver and decided to leave the hospital, he continued to provide supervision throughout the duration of my internship. However, instead of meeting in clinic rooms and administrative offices, we met for supervision on college campuses, respective homes, pubs, and parks. Our ability to connect outside the clinical setting was a unique opportunity to fuse professional development with other interests driven by personal, political, and sometimes unidentified motives. As our relationship evolved from a mentor–mentee nature to that of running buddies and philosophical conversationalists, I sought a deeper level of direction from Michael. I shared stories of traveling alone and working abroad for much of my twenties, and I confided in Michael my apprehensions associated with starting a career, buying a home, and finding myself in a long-term relationship.

At the same time, I actually felt as though I was providing something valuable in return. Michael openly shared difficult memories of losing his dad and reflected on his position as the youngest sibling in a large family. He also shared a distant goal to complete a marathon that was derailed by injury. I encouraged Michael to run with me and provided a training plan to steadily increase distance while allowing for ample recovery. I still felt as though Michael was providing much more than I could in return, but I cherished the notion of helping him complete a marathon and congratulating him at the finish line.

Michael: After John completed his MSW, we began to run together as I continued to supervise him toward his LCSW after he was hired at the hospital. While our supervision became less and less about our fathers over time, it was definitely the common experience that brought us closer together, despite the 22-year age difference. While John continued to develop as a social worker and as a human being, I had a ringside seat at his transformation. I was able to challenge and push him, and he did the same for me. This relationship culminated when I was honored to be the officiant at John's wedding to his bride, Meghan, a defining experience for me that was memorable and meaningful.

John: Five years after meeting Michael and embarking on an internship that would impact both our lives, his insight and guidance far surpassed professional supervision. A level of closeness that I never anticipated reached its peak when Michael agreed to officiate my wedding. In true mentorship fashion, he required that Meghan and I examine our commitment to one another with Michael and his wife, Lisa. We spent the 2 weeks leading up to the wedding delving into the depths of our relationship and tackling difficult questions. Working intimately with Michael and Lisa helped us incorporate the meaning we hoped for during our ceremony. This was evidenced by Michael's personal account of becoming close with us and watching our relationship grow for 5 years. To gain an engaged mentor from an internship could be considered lucky, but to earn a lifelong friend is the result of candid openness, consistent deep connection, and maybe just a bit of fate.

Michael: No one ever teaches us how to be a mentor. While there are certainly professional ethics and guidelines that we should all follow, we should be open to the meaning and exchange that can occur during these mentoring relationships. If we are fortunate, we cross paths with those individuals who make us professionally and personally better people. I can certainly say that was the case for John and me.

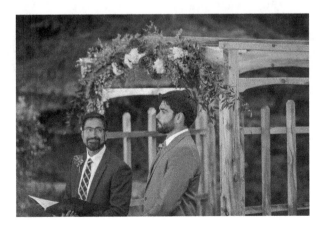

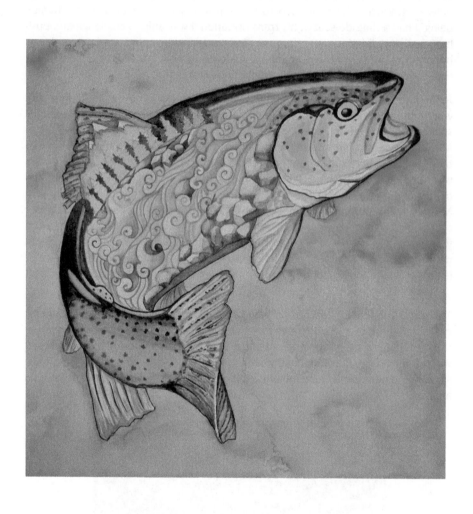

Reflection on Teachers and Mentors: A Parable

Juli Larsen

Long ago, on a high mountain, a small stream began to flow down the mountainside. It flowed, gathering energy and water from the many melting snowfields. The small stream trickled into a larger creek, sharing what it had to offer to the strength and direction of the creek. The creek welcomed the flow. As the creek journeyed downhill, the water gathered heat from the earth, and small plants and animals began to live and thrive within the water.

Among these animals was a newly hatched river trout. The trout was anxious to travel to the larger rivers down in the valley. The trout would skim in and out of the creek's small current, searching for a sign of the larger river. The young trout was eager to learn about the rivers that lie ahead.

The creek was a place of nurturance for the young trout. The flow was slow, the pathway manageable. The trout moved with curiosity and energy, building strength and learning about the world around him.

Soon the creek bid goodbye to the trout as it emptied into a narrow river at the base of the mountain. The river trout anxiously explored his new surroundings. The river was warmer, swifter, and wider. There was more plant life here, more colorful rocks, and there were other fish traveling toward the larger rivers.

The trout watched as the other fish would navigate into the currents, selecting a current that spoke of the larger rivers ahead. Some currents tossed and turned, but were noise unto themselves and the trout could not hear the call of the larger river while near these currents. Some currents appeared content with their slowly swirling flow and undetermined destination.

The trout searched and waited until he found a river current who was listening to the call of the larger river. The trout asked if he could join her in the journey to the larger river. The current was pleased. The trout asked the current about the journey for she had traveled in many rivers and experienced all kinds of waters.

The current told the trout about the riverbed and how it would invite the water to flow in various ways. "When the riverbed narrows, we flow quickly and you will feel excitement and fear, but you are safe. When the water swells wide, we will slow and you will explore and rest." The trout trusted the current and moved through her waters with ease.

The riverbed began to narrow, and the trout felt the stronger, faster pull of the current. The trout yielded to that pull, and the river became a swirl of color around him as he skimmed through the water at incredible speeds. The small trout felt excited and fearful, but safe.

The water began to pool, and the current slowed once more. The trout had more independence here and developed his muscles, "thick shoulders" as some call it; sometimes pushing against the current, sometimes swimming outside of the current. Together they talked of the larger river, and she taught the young trout about the difficulties ahead. "We will come to boulders and logs in the river that create a spinning current. The water will be loud and cloudy with much commotion. You may want to retreat, but you are a trout, and you hear the call of the larger river, so you will find a way through. I will go before you and you can follow."

The current taught the trout to "hold station," to stay still and observe, to prepare before making a run through the turbulent water. The trout practiced. The trout trusted.

Soon, the current began to pull harder, the water became cloudy, and the noise was growing. The trout could see the boulders ahead, and a fallen tree blocking some of the river. The trout began to worry, to doubt. The current stayed close. The trout "held station" and observed. The current moved into the swirling commotion and with an encouraging tug, invited the trout to follow.

With a quick breath of courage, the trout yielded to the current and was swept up into the furious pace of the river's flow. Channeling its inner strength and ability, the trout angled toward the vortex, flexing its body away from the swirling mass of energy, and with one instinctual movement, the trout snapped its body toward the vortex, harvesting energy and power, streaking past at speeds it had never known before.

Breathless and amazed, the trout shot out and met the waiting current on the other side. The trout told her about his terror and his newfound ability. She replied, "You are a trout. You have gifts to use. Use them well. There will be many chances to use your gifts in the larger rivers." The current smiled upon the trout. The trout felt hopeful.

The larger river was louder now. Soon the current and the trout would empty into the larger river. Around the next corner, the river's flow began to deepen, to slow, to merge. They had arrived at the next river, a larger river. With one more pull, the current encouraged the trout into the larger river. The trout darted around exploring the new river. The current explained, "Now you must hear the call of the next larger river. When you hear the call, find the current that is also listening to that same call and flow on."

The young trout, now stronger and more experienced, paused and humbly thanked the current for her influence, guidance, and encouragement. The trout swam off ahead, and the current flowed on, steady, listening for the sound of the next river and waiting for the fish that would follow her on the journey.

This is a story that we play out every day of our lives. We are mentored, or we are mentoring. We are the trout or we are the current. At times, we encourage the upward development of another and in other situations we are the ones who yield to wise influence. An appreciation for both roles benefits our journey downstream.

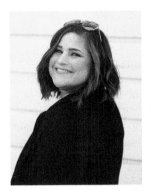

Cameron Froude is a licensed therapist and founder of Bliss In Being Family Therapy, Inc. She completed her PhD in Human Development and Family Studies at the University of Connecticut and a Certificate of Advanced Specialization in Family Medicine Education from the University of Colorado School of Medicine. Dr. Froude assists health and educational systems in mental health integration and supports trauma survivors and their family members in somatic based therapy. Her past times include creative writing and connecting with friends and family.

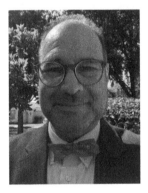

Jeffrey Ring is a clinical health psychologist in Los Angeles. He conducts projects related to health equity and justice, coaching teams and leaders for enlightened leadership, practitioner resilience and vitality, and behavioral health integration. He is the first author of the book, Curriculum for Culturally Responsive Care: The Step-by-Step Guide for Cultural Competence Training.

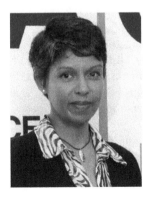

Ajantha Jayabarathan is a family doctor and Director of Coral Shared-Care Health Center, located in Halifax, Nova Scotia, Canada. She completed her medical training at the University of Western Ontario in 1989 and her residency in Family Medicine at Dalhousie University in 1991. She has been writing a column for the Chronicle Herald since 2016, and has also contributed through appearances on television and radio since 1996. Her past times include activities that explore the mind, body and spirit.

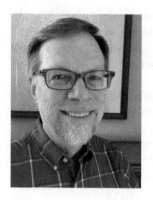

David B. Seaburn PhD, LMFT, was an Assistant Professor, Psychiatry and Family Medicine, at the University of Rochester School Medical Center. In Psychiatry he was Director of the Family Therapy Training Program; in Family Medicine he coordinated the Psychosocial Medicine Rotation. Seaburn was a pioneer in the Medical Family Therapy field, co-authoring Family-oriented Primary Care and Models of Collaboration. Seaburn has also written seven novels and is a retired Presbyterian minister.

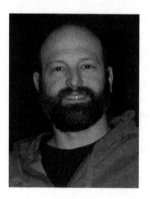

Andrew S. Valeras DO, MPH, FAAFP, is the Associate Program Director for the Dartmouth Hitchcock Leadership Preventive Medicine Residency. He completed his Doctor of Osteopathy from Midwestern University and post graduate training NH Dartmouth Family Medicine Residency in Concord NH where he still lives and works with his wife Aimee (The better writer). Andy enjoys being outdoors with his family and Atticus (named for the famous literary character) their Bernese mountain dog.

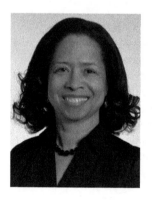

Kathryn Fraser PhD, is the Behavioral Medicine Coordinator at the Halifax Health Family Medicine Residency. She completed a doctorate in Counseling Psychology in 1994 and has published in the areas of counseling skills for family physicians as well as the role of awe in psychotherapy. Outside work, she enjoys yoga, needlework, exploring Florida's parks, and all things food related.

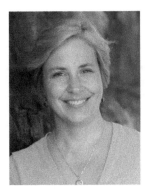

Claudia Worrell Allen PhD, ABPP, is the Director of Behavioral Science in the Department of Family Medicine at the University of Virginia. She completed a doctorate in Psychology at the University of Virginia in 1996 and a juris doctor at Yale Law School in 1986. Outside of work she enjoys stewarding a Little Free Library, attempting to train a therapy dog, and spending time with family in Maine.

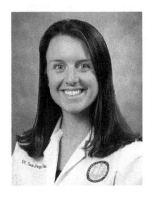

Laura E. Sudano PhD, LMFT, is the Associate Director for Integrated Behavioral Health and behavioral science faculty at the University of California San Diego. She completed a doctorate in Human Development with emphasis in Marriage and Family Therapy at Virginia Polytechnic Institute and State University (Virginia Tech) in 2015. Outside of work she enjoys being active with her family and friends.

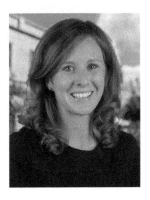

Florencia Lebensohn-Chialvo PhD, is an Assistant Professor in the Marital and Family Therapy Program at the University of San Diego. She completed her doctorate in Clinical Psychology at the University of Arizona in 2015. Outside of work, she looks forward to time with family and friends and traveling abroad, whenever possible.

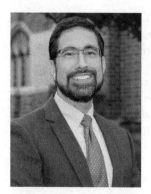

Michael M. Talamantes LCSW, is a Clinical Associate Professor at the Graduate School of Social Work (GSWW) at the University of Denver. He completed his Master of Science in Social Work from the University of Texas at Arlington in 1992. Outside of work, he enjoys running, spending time with his wife & adult children and following the Dallas Cowboys.

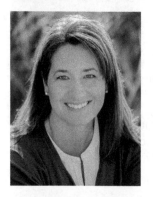

Juli Larsen BS, C-MI, is a meditation instructor in Grand Junction, CO. She completed her under-graduate work at Brigham Young University, majoring in Health Promotions. She enjoys philosophical con-versations with her husband, discussing good books with her 5 children, and spending precious quiet time swimming and gardening.

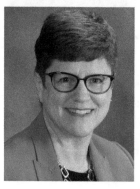

Colleen T. Fogarty MD, MSc, FAAFP, is the William Rocktaschel Professor and Chair of the Department of Family Medicine at the University of Rochester Department of Family Medicine. She earned her MD degree at the University of Connecticut School of Medicine in 1992. Dr. Fogarty is considered an expert in writing 55-word stories and using them as an edu-cational tool for self-reflection. She has published many of these stories, poetry, and narrative essays in several journals.

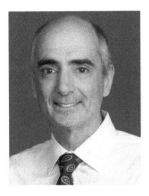

John Spangler MD, is a Professor of Family Medicine, Psychiatry and Epidemiology at Wake Forest School of Medicine. He has a strong interest in addiction medicine and obesity as well as the epidemiology, prevention and cessation of tobacco use. He leads two opioid addiction clinics and tobacco cessation group and individual counseling sessions. An avid writer, he has widely published in the medical literature and academic and lay press. His greatest passion is his family of six children and two grandchildren and he also enjoys reading and ethnic cooking.

Reference

Budman, S. H., Demby, A., Redondo, J. P., Hannan, M., Feldstein, M., Ring, J., et al. (1988). Comparative outcome in time-limited individual and group psychotherapy. *International Journal of Group Psychotherapy, 38*(1), 63–86.

Our Patients and Ourselves

Electronic supplementary material The online version of this chapter (https://doi.org/10.
1007/978-3-030-46274-1_3) contains supplementary material, which is available to authorized
users.

R. Reitz et al. (eds.), *Connections in the Clinic*,
https://doi.org/10.1007/978-3-030-46274-1_3

The Things They Gave Me

Colleen T. Fogarty

Hand-toile-painted box...
Vintage baseball cards,
Souvenirs from home—
Pottery Cuban ashtray,
Albanian pastoral painting framed in amber,
Black ball gown with matching jewelry—

I hope you like it—not expensive, in Vietnam, things are cheap.

The best gift, words of confidence, and trust:

I tell everybody, my doctor is **so** nice!

Their gratitude connecting with mine.

What Do You Know? Start There

Amy L. Davis and Lucy Graham

This narrative is about a Cora Indian living in rural Colorado. The Cora are a tribe of indigenous people in the Sierra Madre Occidental Mountains of Western Mexico. Because of the remoteness of their communities, they have kept their own tribal identities, culture, and language. This narrative combines the prose of a primary care HIV specialist (ALD) with an italicized poem written by her nurse (LG).

As the work day comes to a close, I take a breath, slow my pace and allow the effort of the day to pass over me as a deep exhalation. The impact of this day pushes to the front of my consciousness, demanding reconciliation. On this day, a young Cora Indian from rural Mexico named "Francisco" has made the decision to terminate all treatment for his advanced AIDS and its complications from which he is suffering. My time and conversations with Francisco replay over and over; I feel uneasy.

I first met Francisco many years ago when he arrived in western Colorado as an immigrant farm worker. He had a radiant smile which helped to ease our communication woes. He was nearly deaf from syphilis, spoke the native Cora dialect as his first language and rudimentary Spanish as a second language. Initially, he would take the bus from a little town an hour away to engage in care.

He had been very ill and recently hospitalized with a compromised immune system. He was wary of us, yet also wanted to please us. He would nod vigorously that he wanted treatment, but then would leave only to cast aside our advice. We worked hard to overcome the communication barriers. We frequently used technology to amplify sound as well as a pair of interpreters—one from Cora to Spanish and the second from Spanish to English.

Other than a reported brother who roamed somewhere in the desert southwest, Francisco had no known family or friends. His social services case manager and our clinic staff had become his family, his advocacy; we rallied to try to assist him to better health. Still, he would disappear from care for months at a time. His health deteriorated.

Recently, his case manager had found him a place to stay in town and she enveloped him in a package of services. Dutifully, he came to the clinic, always smiling. He never said much. But I was hopeful that with assistance, his health might improve.

Today's meeting with him was a home visit. His case manager had called me. Francisco was ill and losing weight. She had discovered, he was not taking any of his medications. Using our awkward combination of amplification devices and interpreters, I asked him about his medications. He informed me that he would no longer take any medications for HIV or antibiotics to protect him from complications. I held his hand and tried to understand what he was thinking. "Why?" I asked. "Please tell me about this." He responded, "The Black Gods have told me not to take the pills." He would say no more.

> I held his hand and tried to understand what he was thinking. "Why?" I asked. "Please tell me about this." He responded, "The Black Gods have told me not to take the pills." He would say no more.

The Cora believe that to furnish outsiders with any information might then cause illness or death because of the displeasure of the deities. They believe that humans must cooperate with the gods to maintain the order of the cosmos. Francisco seemed neither anxious nor fearful, but still I worried. He was choosing a preventable death, in essence a passive suicide. Does he have capacity to make this decision? Is he depressed? Is he psychotic? Or is his decision truly congruent with his spiritual and cultural beliefs. How can I possibly tell the difference given our barriers to communication and our lack of family availability. What is my responsibility to him now?

> I enter the exam room and my mind flashes
> to the thousand-piece puzzle I'm working on at home.
> I have found all the border pieces, the easy part,
> by picking out the flat edges and corners.
>
> My real work then begins in a contained, but empty rectangle,
> a picture of the solution ever-present.
> It may not be quick or easy to finish, but I am confident and patient,
> and I have usually found success.
>
> This day, with this patient,
> I feel as if I've been given a borderless, monochromatic puzzle to solve.
> I am unsure, anxious, and find a starting point more than elusive.
> I am so out of my comfort zone.

Then I remember what my mother always said
when I fretted over a difficult problem growing up:
"What do you know?
Start there."

I know very little,
but I know how to care about the lived experiences of others.
Instead of trying to solve him,
I start to try and understand him.

I hear what he says, even though I don't speak his language.
Our shared space is peaceful, calm, and unrelenting.
He transforms my practice from problem-focused
to one of discovery and intentional patient-centeredness.

I wave good-bye as I leave the room, knowing I will never see him again.

As I sat in my chair in the dim late afternoon light, staring out of the glass windows, I felt a hand on my shoulder. My psychologist colleague, John, sat beside me, and all of my angst and doubt spilt out, as I recounted my story. He looked at me intently for a moment. He said, "I'm going to challenge you, if I may." I nodded. He continued, "For some, death is not a thing to be feared nor avoided. It may not be an end. I might ask that you put aside your own worry about his choice and your instinct to treat him, and be at peace with what he is requesting."

I thought about my conversation with John much that evening and would occasionally think about Francisco's decision for years to come. We respected and honored Francisco's decision. We were never able to find any family, but those of us who knew and cared about him supported him as best we could. He never seemed to suffer nor waiver. He peacefully left us two weeks later.

The Indignity of Dying

Alice Yuxi Lu

Her husband had arrived at the trauma bay minutes earlier—pupils unresponsive, no respirations, no pulses, no cardiac activity seen on ultrasound. Barely after he was pronounced dead—the first death pronouncement I had ever seen—they announced the second patient: same motor vehicle collision, en route, ETA 10 min.

As she was wheeled into the room, her skin jiggled with every downstroke of the automated CPR machine. The rhythmic click of the machine sounded an underlying beat to the physicians and nurses whirling around her as if in a complicated ballet. I stood there clinging to the edge of this well-rehearsed dance watching in awe and growing trepidation.

On TV, dead people are always pale, white, and bloodless, as if they had been dipped in a vat of flour. But her skin had a waxy sheen under the fluorescent lights. Yellow—on another person I would have called it "jaundiced"—a term we learned early in medical school describing the yellowing of the skin due to excess bilirubin. They never taught us what to call the yellowing of the skin during death.

They also never taught us about the indignity of dying. In the trauma bay, our goal is to keep the patient alive and stabilized—and we will do anything to achieve it. We cut off clothing to look for injuries—exposing everything under the harsh bright lights. We stick needles into any opening we can get—arms, feet, groin—to pump in fluids and blood. We break ribs. We cut open and thrust hands into the chest cavity to keep a barely quivering heart pumping. We do all these to save a patient's life. Sometimes, to justify what we are doing to our patients, we have to push to the back of our minds that this is a human life; we intentionally forget that they are more than the flesh we are cutting into or body parts we are manipulating. But standing there, it hit me all of a sudden that this was a woman with plans and hopes and dreams—all because of a single sneaker.

From where I was standing, I had a perfect view of her feet, sticking out from the cluster of physicians surrounding her. One foot was bare, but on the other was a familiar green and teal sneaker. The same sneaker I would have seen if I looked down, past the blue protective gown and scrubs, enclosing my own feet. Was this woman a runner like me? Did she go on a morning run, as I had, wearing these sneakers with scuff marks on the side? Was this woman planning on going on a hike with her husband in these sneakers with dirt embedded in the soles? What else have those sneakers brought this woman through? What else in life have they walked through together? That brief glimpse reminded me of her humanity, the memory of which will be forever kept alive for me by this green and teal sneaker.

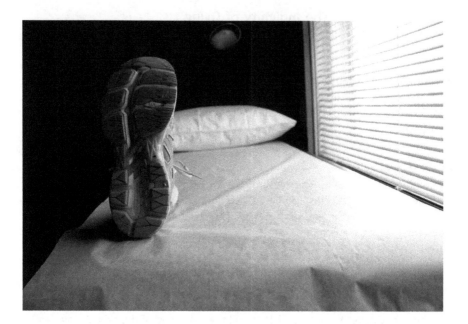

Leading by Example: A Story About a Woman with Parkinson's Disease

Jennifer Hodgson

Sylvia was one of those compassionate, intelligent, talented, and strong female leaders who other women stand on the shoulders of with pride. Our relationship was multifaceted, going from co-leaders of a local support group to close friends in over a decade's time. An example of her impact on my life was when my oldest daughter was born. She knew something I did not, that my daughter like her would find life and light in art. She bought her a beautifully painted child-sized table and chairs at which to sit and create her mini masterpieces. Little did she know, my daughter would grow up to be a gifted artist just like her. True leaders have that remarkable gift of insight and know-how to bring out the talents in others. Sylvia had it in abundance.

When Sylvia McCreary was in her 60s, she was stricken with Parkinson's disease. It stole her beautiful voice, effortless smile, long strong body, and perfect penmanship, but it did not waiver her ability to communicate and lead. She expected the best out of everyone around her, but more importantly herself.

Sylvia was an accomplished organist who played for her church every week. People all over eastern North Carolina requested her for weddings, funerals, and other important events. Sadly, her diagnosis of Parkinson's disease compromised her ability to maneuver the organ and play to her standard of excellence. However, if you were lucky enough she would share recordings of her cherished performances. The sound processed through an old cassette tape player just added to the charm. When Parkinson's disease stole her identity as an organist, she adopted a new one. She initiated the first Parkinson's support group in eastern North Carolina with a local physical therapist, Jean Lambert.

When I met Sylvia, a few years after she started the support group, she was still driving and her disease had only started to impact her freedom of movement. She dealt with her tremor through medication and refused to allow her symptoms to interfere with the joy she felt when with her children, grandchildren, church community, and enjoying her emerging interests.

> While her body was being ravaged by her disease, her activism and commitment to bringing hope to others strengthened.

She discovered a new talent as she stepped away from the organ; she was an amazing watercolor painter. She painted with precision and could capture life as she saw it: beautiful, colorful, and always vibrant. She would pick up a paintbrush and inexplicably her tremor would quell. One of my favorite pieces she painted, that appeared on a stand at the base of her hospice bed, was of a red wagon filled with colorful flowers. She started painting to help raise funds for the support group and even held a session for the members of the support group to learn to paint. She wanted them to know that Parkinson's was not the end but the beginning. She wanted people to discover the hidden talents that also live inside of them. The last piece she did was of my three children. I did not know until later how she struggled to complete it, fighting fatigue with each stroke of her brush. She honored her commitments to a fault.

As co-facilitators of the Parkinson's support group, we worked together for years designing meeting agendas, planning psychoeducational talks, fundraising, and hosting local conferences. Sylvia wanted the group to be strength-based and not doom and gloom. She wanted better resources for those living east of Interstate 95, the roadway the separates the thriving industrial centers from the vanishing farming communities. The closest Parkinson's Center for Excellence (known for innovations in Parkinson's treatment and research) was almost 2 hours away so she also championed for a local neurologist to develop expertise in Parkinson's care so our members did not have to drive so far for effective treatment. While her body was being ravaged by her disease, her activism, and commitment to bringing hope to others strengthened. She never stopped leading even after she passed the microphone to the other support group facilitators. When her voice was inaudible on the phone, another devastating symptom of Parkinson's disease, her husband, Gene would call with her requests and ideas for the group. It was ironic how her ability to lead strengthened as her speaking voice weakened.

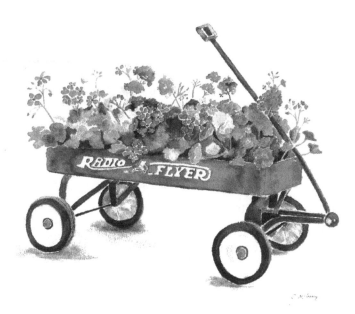

Sylvia was a natural leader. Those of us privileged to be around her were her foot soldiers. We were extensions of her voice, hands, arms, and legs as her Parkinson's disease progressed, and the medications she was given decreased in their effectiveness. We worked together like a fluid and gentle wave.

It was hard saying no to Sylvia.

How could you say no to someone who was doing this work, not just to benefit her own quality of life, but also the lives of others? Admittedly, I did miss a few meetings when I had a lot to do at work or when my children needed me to just be still at home. She always gave me space and grace. She knew leaders too sometimes needed to step back to move forward. Sylvia taught me a lot about the importance of self-care and putting family first. She invested in me as a person and that made me want to invest right back.

After Sylvia died, we were faced with the unspeakable decision of whether or not to continue the support group. The other facilitator who started the group with her, Jean Lambert, struggled to continue in her leadership role. The grief was intense. I knew if the group was going to continue, I needed help.

A Speech and Language Pathology faculty member, Balaji Rangarathnam, PhD, who was interested in Parkinson's disease and one of his faculty colleagues, Kathrin Rothermich, PhD, agreed to join the team. Both new in their faculty roles, they have grown in their investment with the group in a way Sylvia would have liked. They jumped right in and helped take on roles of agenda planning, writing grants, designing research studies, and giving presentations to the members. We learned to rotate many of these responsibilities amongst ourselves, careful not to burn any one of us out. Several caregivers, Patsy Cooke and Patricia Rawls, also stepped into leadership roles and helped to manage the administrative tasks of the group which included registering new members, setting up for the meetings, and calling members when meeting reminders were needed. We all tried, and continue to try, to lead by the example that Sylvia set.

Sylvia would be proud that the group she started 20 years ago is still in existence.

She taught me so many invaluable lessons about what it means to remain devoted to something. Sylvia appreciated that I was a mother and a full-time professor and as I said, supported me in stepping back from time to time. However, she would not allow me to use being too busy as an excuse for too long. She didn't. When she hurt, she was there. When she struggled to move, she asked for help. When she lacked the voice to speak, she handed the microphone to the next person. The group was never about how great she was or what she accomplished in her role, but her belief in the group and what it was created to do.

Relationships were central to her leadership style and she invested in them. This made us want to contribute even more to the work she began. When we disagreed, we talked it out. When we drifted apart due to competing responsibilities, she gently reigned us in. I think I still hear her voice at times activating me to do something for the group that needs to be done. When I need a boost, one of her paintings that is around my office and home will catch my eye. At those moments, I tell myself, "If Sylvia could do it, you can too!" I learned from her that you invest in the people around you and you need to lead by example. You do not give up on the journey but rather modify how you complete it. That is how you get things done!

The Complaint

Mark P. Knudson

Thirteen minutes! The nurse who listened to the patient and called me said it may be a record. "Thirteen minutes is too long to send you the whole audio-file," she shared, "but I can tell you some of the concerns."

The nurse then listed the series of patient grievances starting with my refusal to see Ellen last week. "Ellen," a 52-year-old patient, left out the fact that she had been 35 min late. Instead, the complaint meandered from present to past and encompassed a host of alleged transgressions.

"You never looked at my draining left ear 3 years ago," Ellen complained on the taped message, followed by "Jack's Hospice referral should have been sooner." She jumped from her hair to her feet in the complaints, found issues as far back as 19 years ago, and listed at least 12 medications I should have prescribed along with 7 diseases that I had missed.

The next 2 days were filled with anger, frustration, remorse, more anger, and a sense of deflation. The fact that I had not slept soundly recently didn't help. But each Monday when morning came, the cycle started again. Morning clinic with a packed schedule. Patients that weren't mine squeezed in, with seemingly endless festering problems. Then patients either arrived late or if they arrived on time they had to wait in long lines at the reception. And if one patient no-showed a 9:30 appointment (false hope of a short break), their 9:30 spot would be filled at 9:47 by another patient who expected to be seen even though they could not get into the clinic till 10:10, leaving me with three patients—the 9:45 patient who showed up 20 min late, the 10:00 patient who was just getting in a room because they had to empty their bladder first, and this new patient added to the schedule.

Noontime was swept away by the never-ending stream of patients left from the morning, and when I finally got down to the educational lunch meeting, the talk was done and the students had finished the last bit of food, leaving only a few shards of iceberg lettuce wilting in a plastic bowl, and some chicken pie crust that was "too small for the other Who's mouses."

Precepting in the afternoon was a frantic mix of trying to teach residents in the clinic while refilling narcotic scripts for Dr. Hardassy while she was in Hawaii, re-ordering the breast Ultrasound for the resident who didn't know which of the 42 "Breast US" orders were the right one, and calling the insurance company about the Chest CT that had to be pre-approved even though the short of breath tobacco-smoking patient was coughing up blood and had a mass on the Chest X-ray.

I finally got home to my South Beach diet dinner (much needed since I had gained 10 lbs in the last year, but not as comforting.) This was followed by nightly charting on a computer that was slow to start up and sometimes shut off of its own accord.

Two days after I'd received the "record setting" complaint, I was scheduled to meet with Ellen. I was anxious about the meeting all day long. Distracted, I forgot to tell anyone about Mr. Baker who showed up at 8:00 AM without an appointment, even though I had asked him to come in. I sent Mrs. Smart to the lab, which didn't work since I had ordered a Chest X-ray and not labs. And the pharmacy called back about a prescription, complaining that my directions didn't make sense (and when I angrily took the message and saw what I had written, I realized that my orders didn't make sense!)

I carved out time to see Ellen off schedule and by the time I went to see her I was pretty shaken. I feared that the anger that triggered this 13-min complaint would bubble over to make this a truly painful appointment. But before I could say much more than "Good afternoon, Mrs. Dempsey," she started to echo the list of complaints. She recounted that I had not seen her when she came to the clinic last week, even if she was very late, and I made her feel guilty about refilling meds, even though she understood that some of the medications weren't good for her. But one by one, these complaints and others melted into an apology from her, stating that she was sorry that she had called to complain. She started to get teary-eyed when she recalled how I had cared for her for more than 20 years. She remembered how I had taken care of her grandson at that time he was so sick, coming in late at night to see him. And the tears really opened up when she told me how important it was when I came to Jack's funeral 2 years ago.

I flashed back to something I had written that night. It had started in my head as I drove an hour from the rural town where he was buried. I had written about the final hospital visit when he was admitted just days after she had slammed the door on the hospice nurses insisting that he was going to pull through this.

A rhythmic hum of oxygen pumped thru tubes,
Held the room in silence.
I lifted his bloated hand, cold, silent too!
From behind, her gentle sob broke the quiet,
And I hugged her.
17 years, more his Doctor than hers,
We shared the same role of caring for him.
A role that now was ending,
For both of us, in silence.

Today, she laughed about how I was the only doctor who knew Jack. She talked about how she had loved him, hated him, and been scared of him till the day that she realized that he became a mean-spirited shit when he was drinking. But she also remembered realizing that she had the upper hand when he was drunk, and had managed to deck him quite cleanly a time or two. And she got quiet when she told me, in spite of all his meanness and violence, that she missed the old son of a bitch a lot, and she was grateful that I was there for him. And today, she said, she was grateful that I was there for her.

And in spite of a 13-min grievance call, I realized that I was grateful, too.

King's Story

Jennifer L. Ayres

"You don't recognize me, do you?" A heavily tattooed, multi-pierced young man sat next to me on the bench outside of the Mexican food restaurant where I take my children for breakfast most Saturday mornings. The overpowering cologne did not mask the smoke underneath it. I took my eyes away from my 7-year-old sons and glanced in the old eyes of the young man. I flipped quickly through my mental collage of children I've seen who now are young adults. My search yielded no results. He grinned at me. "You said I'm the only person you'll ever meet with my name. It's me, Dr. Ayres. King."

* * *

I met "King" and his 50-year-old, cousin-turned-guardian when his primary care physician referred him for therapy evaluation. He was one of the well-child checks that turned complicated once the physician began to delve into social history. And his social history was complicated, starting with his name. His father chose the name King because "that way my boy will always have respect." I met him twice in the 5 years I worked with his son, due to his repeat incarcerations for drug-related charges. His mother abandoned the father and their three children for a life that she predicted would be easier and had voluntarily relinquished her parental rights long before I met King. His older sister, at 10, exhibited early signs of antisocial personality, and a younger brother, age 6, showed signs of precocious, manipulative behavior. King was inattentive, hyperactive, noncompliant, and carried the always suspicious affect of a child unfamiliar with a non-traumatic life.

He and his cousin sat on the couch in my office. His feet dangled above the floor and kicked the back of the couch. He avoided eye contact. His cousin was angry and overwhelmed by him and the generations of family chaos that he represented. I brought approximately 10 years of experience to that initial evaluation and I was overwhelmed by the road ahead of this 8-year-old boy who carried the weight of broken ancestors. He had worked with several therapists by that point in his young life and I asked what he hoped I could do for him.

"I don't want to be so mad anymore."

Over the course of five years, we worked on his anger as chaos swirled around him. His father repeated his "incarceration-release-promises" cycle twice. His older sister was sent to residential treatment. His younger brother went inpatient following multiple contacts with the county's mental health emergency response team for conduct dis-

> If I breathe deeply enough and close my eyes, I smell the cologne that never quite masked what it was trying to cover.

ordered behavior and suicidal ideation. King, however, got better. He, his cousin, and I decided that he was ready for a break from therapy and they agreed to call me if they needed my help in the future.

And I didn't see him for seven years until that morning he sat next to me on the bench.

* * *

I hugged him tightly, absorbing his heavy cologne. He updated me on his family. His father was very sick, in the hospital with end-stage medical issues of some unspecified type. His brother and sister were living their life course. His cousin was doing well. King was working at the Mexican food restaurant as a host and was in the process of completing a GED. He aspired to become a server once he turned 21, 1 year away. He seated us, hugged me, and walked back to the podium. The young boy who held so little power now was a grown man with a throne.

When we were leaving, he hugged me again. He held tightly, reluctant to pull away. I loosened my hold, but he held on. I patted his back and had a brief flashback to a similar moment that occurred when he was about 10, a decade earlier. He was crying because his father was going back to jail for drug possession. Again. "But he promised" was all his voice that was too old for his age could manage. I moved from my chair to sit next to him on the couch, an effort to show him that I was present and he was not going to carry this pain and burden alone. As he moved closer and hugged me, I wondered how many people hugged this hurting little boy. I had read an article about how many daily hugs a person needed to be emotionally connected and mentally healthy. And I wondered if he would ever get enough hugs to compensate for the ones he hadn't received.

He pulled away and looked at me. "Do you still have that couch?" I nodded. He smiled. "Do you still have those games?" I nodded. "Good. I liked the games." I smiled at him. He turned to my sons. "You're really lucky." I hugged him one last time and absorbed cologne that stayed with me for the rest of the day. As we walked to the car, I heard him say to his coworker, "That's my therapist."

* * *

For about 3 months, I saw King at least once a week at that restaurant. He knew my children by name and they called him King and my "friend." Every time we saw him, he shared me another story about a recent happening that told me the chaos of the ancestors had not escaped him, despite our best effort. One morning he approached us and told me he had really good news. He had been waiting for me to arrive so he could tell me. His girlfriend was pregnant and he was excited to be a dad. He wanted to be a good dad and someone "my kid is proud of." I said that sounded like a great goal.

After several Saturday mornings of not seeing him, I asked one of the servers about him. She said that he didn't work there anymore and that she wasn't sure what happened.

I last saw him almost a year ago and wonder what happened. Was the chaos of the ancestors too strong of a pull that the monotony of sustained employment and a schedule couldn't counterbalance? Is he incarcerated? If so, why? His child must be an infant now. What patterns does King carry into parenting? What patterns were broken? How many hugs does he receive a day and how does that contribute to the inability to extricate himself from the claws of the chaos?

My sons are now older than he was that first afternoon he sat on my couch with his cousin. They are hugged more often than the current daily recommendation. What chaos will they avoid by that fact alone?

"That's my therapist." A supervisor once told me that after someone becomes your patient, you will always be that person's therapist. It is a role that is never finished. If I breathe deeply enough and close my eyes, I smell the cologne that never quite masked what it was trying to cover.

The Pain Beyond the Pain

Kathryn Warren Hart

They say the eyes are the pathway to the soul
but I'm a dentist and look to the mouth

A toddler in pigtails, dirt under fingernails
right cheek swollen, eye half-winking at me
Life isn't fun enough for a full wink
Abscessed before it even had a chance
Mom says she complained of a toothache, "Just a few times"

A teenager who won't smile is normal, no?
He has a habit of covering his chin
Mumbles a question about braces
as he pulls his lips down to hide

A college girl, a whip, nervous in the chair
I lay her back and I can see
the damage done by the acid that has
many times
passed through her, melting the insides of her teeth
Fragile and translucent now, like thin glass
…like her

A man now, early 30s,
tattoos on his temples, masseter muscles flexing,
shifting, uneasy
decay along the gumline of every remaining tooth.
He blames prison
    his upbringing
    his genes
He wants to know what I can prescribe

A baby, just 10 months old,
brought by foster-mom
She's worried the baby has no teeth.
not eating well, fussy
      Oh but there are teeth, I mean, there were...
      just root stubs now, covered by swollen gums

An elderly woman from Assisted Living, accompanied by a caretaker
She smiles wide showing dry gums, scratches her boob, curses.
I like her
the woman's son wants her to have dentures.
      ...flushed the last pair.
"Yes, she eats just fine"
The old woman giggles
      but I can hear the cry of the son who misses his mother,
      before dementia
He's crying, "I'm in pain"

I see all these mouths
All this pain beyond the pain

For my part, I remember to breathe calmly
set my teeth,
smile gently

I hope my smile says
I recognize your pain
I want to help you
Let's move forward together now.

Practicing Kindness: One Incrementalist's Approach

Justin H. McCarthy

I first met "Gina" 2 years into one of her several forays into homelessness. I was a first-year resident and she was a late addition to what had already been an exhausting (and admittedly) impersonal call day for me on our hospital's inpatient teaching service. She had presented to the ER for sores on the back of her hand, which she was convinced were brown recluse bites. Homelessness and 40-plus years of hard living showed in her matted hair, cracked lips, leathered skin, and missing front incisors. It had also damaged her psyche and made her mistrusting of others. Rather than stay at a shelter, Gina preferred to "camp" by the Colorado River and ride her bicycle around town, which she strapped down with all of her belongings.

But I wasn't admitting Gina for bug bites; after all, we don't even have brown recluse spiders in this part of the state, a fact Gina quickly dismissed by a theory that they migrated here in rail cars. Rather, she was being admitted for a blood sugar ten times normal levels, which was found, incidentally, with routine blood work. Gina seemed neither interested in my medical knowledge nor her new diagnosis of diabetes. She simply wanted reassurance that her hand would be okay. Her irrational and odd thinking wasn't so much frustrating to me as it was intriguing. I knew I needed to convince her to remain in the hospital. Yet, I struggled to form an argument that would convince her to stay.

Having run a homeless clinic during my 4 years of medical school, I knew how often mental illness and substance use issues went together. I also appreciated how lacking basic necessities could color a patient's priorities to be different than mine and the medical establishment's. I immediately started applying this narrative to Gina and was not surprised to read that she had a history of alcohol use disorder leading to liver cirrhosis. It was during one of her follow-up visits with the gastroenterologist that she was diagnosed with exocrine pancreatic insufficiency which led to her diabetes. Gina didn't know anything about diabetes. She was 6 months sober and oddly cavalier about it—as though it

> After initially stating that she would wait for me to get AMA paperwork drafted up, she left unannounced but not before defecating in the front lobby of the hospital.

was no big accomplishment. Even more striking, she was a practicing vegan, which seemed remarkably inconvenient given her current living circumstances and her blood sugar level. Like so many patients, what was important to Gina seemed at odds with bettering her health.

As Gina removed her many layers of clothes for me to perform a physical exam, my heart sank as the extent of her malnutrition revealed itself. Emaciated, weak, and unbalanced, I found myself questioning what good hospitalization would ultimately do her. She seemed to be one foot in the grave. By comparison, the last human I had seen as thin as her was a 92-year-old bed-bound man in the Dominican Republic. He died the next day.

Well, Gina didn't die…and she didn't stay long in the hospital either. After much pleading and bargaining, she agreed to hospitalization. For my part, I had to locate her bike and bring all of her belongings up to her room. Locating her bike took some time and kept me from providing medical care to my other patients. Laden down with her mélange of dirty bags I rode the public elevator up ten floors to her room, catching quite a few looks along the way. Self-conscious about her (my?) baggage, I was concerned about what the hospital staff must think about the new intern who fetched at the beck and call the belongings for his homeless patient. The charge nurse greeted me at the elevator. Whatever they thought of me was overshadowed by what they thought of Gina. In the short time that had passed, she had cursed out one nurse and thrown her plate of food at another.

"You'd better get your patient under control, Dr. McCarthy, or we'll be getting security involved. It's not okay to treat my nurses this way."

I vowed to do my best and arrived at Gina's hospital room in time to witness a flurry of activity just before she demanded to be discharged. I tried explaining why that wasn't safe, then tried reasoning with her, then appealing to her any way that I could. Once again, I found myself marveling at the extra work I was expending to take care of a patient who seemed disinterested in taking care of herself. After initially stating that she would wait for me to get AMA paperwork drafted up, she left unannounced but not before defecating in the front lobby of the hospital.

It wasn't long before Gina returned. I took care of her on four subsequent hospital encounters. I felt strongly that if she had primary care and someone whom she trusted then the hospital, nurses, and food services could be saved from what was becoming weekly admissions. I offered to be "her doctor" and she gladly accepted my offer. As it would turn out, this was a controversial covenant. Her frequent admissions, verbal assaults of female staff, and leaving AMA earned us both a negative reputation.

After a while, Gina did start using insulin but her episodes of high blood sugars quickly became low blood sugars. It was impossible to replicate her diet on the streets while she was in the hospital. As a result, she was repeatedly discharged on insulin regimens, which while appropriate with regular meals in the hospital, tanked her to near-deadly lows on the streets. Her highest blood sugars had been around 1600, but on another of my call days, she came in after being found unresponsive with a blood sugar of 6. Brittle diabetes, like Gina's, is extremely difficult to manage in the best of circumstances. Needless to say, Gina's circumstances were not ideal: homeless, vegan, and living with brain injuries seemed to have made her incapable of following her complicated insulin regimen.

"Would you be willing to stay at a shelter with semi-regular meals?" "No."

"Could you stop being a vegan even for a little bit, while we sort this out?" "No."

"You should be kinder to my female colleagues." "No."

Exasperated and frustrated, the weekly admissions continued. Through trial and error, we gradually selected a regimen that kept her in the 200–400s; essentially a compromise that resulted in a "better-than-nothing" approach.

I remember Gina's first hospital follow-up. Whatever joy I felt at the success of keeping her out of the hospital long enough to come was quickly erased when she showed up 2 hours early, unsettled the waiting room of other patients, and had to be moved to 1 of my 2 rooms to maintain the peace. The last patient of a long day,

I resolved to take a stand. I finally stepped into the room ready to set her straight, when I sensed something was not right.

Gina looked pale.

She was only able to describe the way she felt as, "I ache everywhere. My bones feel like they are breaking." This certainly felt like a turn of events. At a loss and unable to get any other history, I did the unthinkable—I recommended she go to the emergency department. My singular success, ablated.

Serendipitously, I would be heading there shortly for a shift. I quickly wrapped up my notes and readied myself to be ridiculed by the ED staff for sending one of their "frequent flyers" to them for no clear reason. As I passed by her ED room I heard retching, a splatter of something on the floor, and peeked my head in to see the floor and walls painted in blood. Gina lay unconscious, slumped in her hospital gurney. As it turned out, she had a heavily bleeding stomach ulcer from taking the Naproxen I had recommended.

The chaos and uncontrollable circumstances of many patients' lives challenge doctors in ways we are never trained to handle. Being a good physician is less often about getting the right diagnosis or knowing the best treatment and more about recognizing the needs and capabilities of your patient, then tailoring a plan that will work for them. We are taught the ideal and yet rarely get to practice in it. Gina's story, to me, illustrates what Atul Gawande affectionately terms, "work of incrementalists." That is, the glacial work of primary care that slowly and over long periods of time can make the biggest difference.

I fought Gina, pushing my own agenda for a long time. I don't consider myself egotistical but the best practices, evidence-based medicine, and being under constant scrutiny as a doctor-in-training were powerful motivators. It was frustrating to settle for lesser results than what I had expected (and others expected of me, as well). Gina's case felt like a long lesson in humility; one where I abandoned the prestige of my profession and rarely got the results I wanted in return. Ironically, I get to author this narrative as a success story—a "good catch;" simply because on that day, I listened to Gina—even when her description was completely unhelpful. Because we had developed a relationship, I knew her normal and I could tell something was not right. I shudder to think what may have happened if I had not been as attentive or if she had seen someone else at that clinic visit.

Today, thanks to the hard work of our community health workers, Gina now has stable housing, a boyfriend, and is free of admissions for a couple of years. Each time she comes in, she beams one of her toothless smiles, and I right back at her. She brings her logs and her average blood sugar is one of the best in my patient panel. Most of my patients are not like Gina and I truly do not feel like my medical care is what has secreted her success. She needed housing, food security, and a little insulin guidance; but more than anything, Gina needed a relationship with an interdisciplinary staff she trusted. I'd wager all physicians have success stories like Gina. Gina's successes did not subscribe to the conventions I'd imagined. Hers was a frustrating, glacial (almost indiscernible) improvement. It was a story of setbacks and humility without end in sight. I guarantee all physicians have patients who challenge them. Gina's story serves as a reminder to practice kindness and stay vigilant. You never know when that relationship will change dramatically.

Those are the patient–physician relationships that shine light on the holiness of our profession.

The Real Reason the Red Sox Won the World Series

Arnold Goldberg

"Dorothy" laid quietly in the ICU swollen all over. The heart that was always filled with love and caring was now big and flabby, and failing her. Her kidneys were also giving out. So many times, she had dragged herself back from the brink of death. Now it looked bad, really bad. No medications were helping her.

It was early July of 2004. Dorothy had been my patient for over 8 years. There were no children. Now in her early eighties, she had devoted her life to her husband of nearly 60 years. Her husband had suddenly died at home 2 years earlier while Dorothy was in rehab recovering from a small heart attack. Having to go to that nursing home to break the news to her was incredibly difficult. Dorothy's closest relative, a very caring nurse, just couldn't do it. So, her physician went instead. As I drove up to the nursing home I felt tortured like one of those unfortunate military officers driving up in their black sedans to a family to say, "I'm sorry to inform you about your child's death."

I went there to comfort her and myself on that day. I felt like I had failed her. I had cared for her husband also. He died on my watch. I could not fulfill my promise to unite then again when she left the nursing home.

Now Dorothy herself was in the ICU dying and in the middle of the baseball season. You see, besides the doctor–patient relationship, we had another relationship, a contentious one. Dorothy was one of those devoted Red Sox fans, the whole nine yards; the pennants, the hats, and the dreaded curse. Born and bred in the Bronx, I am a true Yankee fan. I bleed pinstripes. My grandfather in the early 1900s rooted for the Highlanders, the ancestors of the Pinstripes. My grandfather passed the passion onto my father and him to me. We watched hundreds of games together from the bleachers. I was an original Bleacher Brat. My dad could never bring himself to pay the $1.25 for a grandstand seat. No, it was 75 cents for a doubleheader and a chance to talk to Mickey Mantle from the centerfield bleachers. Also, it was the only time my dad and I could talk together. I guess that is the power of baseball, to provide the only joyous moments where some fathers and sons can communicate. As I look back on it, I realized that must have been the only time my father could talk to his father, a man affected with bipolar disorder. Baseball will continue to weave this thread throughout generations.

Dorothy's visits to the office in April always began with the optimistic banter about how the Red Sox were going to win it all this year. This will be the year they would finally beat the Yankees. "The Yanks are the best team money could buy!" she would say. I would always point out how the Red Sox were not exactly cheap, having the second highest payroll in baseball.

And so it would go throughout the summertime, until the regular fall time visit when the Yankees would pull ahead and again break her heart and the hearts of Red Sox nation. I thought the 2003 season would have done her in right then and there. Out of her lady-like mouth came the words, "Bleeping Aaron Boone!" as she agonized over this Yankee's extra-inning home run to beat the Red Sox again for the pennant. I just smiled and said, "Wait till next year." I was just humoring her. I knew next year never comes for the Red Sox fans.

So, there we were in the ICU both Dorothy and the Red Sox at Heaven's Gate on that early July day. Dorothy was behind the medical 8 balls and the Red Sox were very far behind the Yankees already. For the Red Sox, there would be another year, but for Dorothy, we both knew that there would be no "wait till next year."

Weekly she said, "Doctor, thanks for everything. I know you really cared about me. I have no regrets I am going to meet up with my husband. Also, I can't wait to give that gentleman, Harry Herbert Frazee, who sold Babe Ruth to the Yankees a good piece of my mind and the Babe, too!" Her niece and I had a good laugh. That was Dorothy, a true Red Sox fan to the end.

Early that morning she peacefully passed away. Her funeral parlor was filled with beautiful flowers. I sat there wishing we had bought her an arrangement that proclaimed "The Red Sox, World Series Champions!!"

That was early July. Some baseball fans point to the trade of Nomar Garciaparra as their season's turning point. Those of us who knew Dorothy knew better. It must have taken just 2 weeks for her to get her audience with the Babe and Harry Frazee. I can just imagine her wagging her finger at them, "Enough is enough you 2! Red Sox nation has suffered enough!" That was late July and in early August the Sox went on a winning tear. The rest is history, all the way to the momentous Game 4 of the American League Championship Series. The Yankees were leading 3 games to none, "Oh well, Dorothy," I said to myself again, "wait until next year." Then came the walk, the steal, the tie, and then the extra-inning home run. I could hear Dorothy say, "Not this time doctor, not this time!" Eight games later the champagne was flowing. The Red Sox were World Champions! I smiled and admitted to myself, well that was for Dorothy. She must have really given it to the Babe.

Two weeks later while I was seeing patients, a delivery came to the office. It was a beautiful plant. Attached to the plant was a card. I opened it up and started to laugh as goose bumps went up to my back. "Dear Dr G, in my Aunt's will included special instructions asked me to bring you this card and plant when the Red Sox beat the Damm Yankees and won the World Series."

Dear Dr G,

If you are reading this then the Red Sox finally won the World Series and beat your Yankees! Hah, Hah, we finally got you!

Best wishes,

Dorothy

I groaned; even from beyond the grave she and the Red Sox got me!

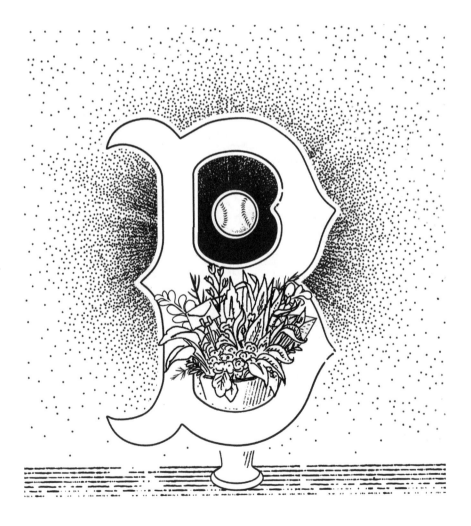

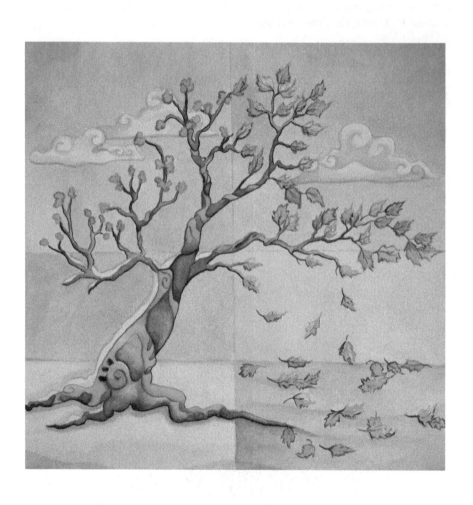

Reflection on Our Patients: Comfort and Growth

Juli Larsen

In the early 1900s, a Chicago Evening Post journalist named Finley Peter Dunne created a famous fictional character, Mr. Doody, who would give voice to his political thoughts and feelings. Mr. Doody notably observed: "The job of the newspaper is to comfort the afflicted and afflict the comfortable."

Every patient that we interact with is a walking version of that same job description: they are here to comfort or afflict us. They usually don't discriminate depending upon the type of day, week, or year we are having. We can usually look at the schedule and breathe relief when we see certain names, trusting that they will show up for the appointment, at the right time, be respectful and attentive, appreciate our offering, and pay on the way out the door. Then there are those names that cause our stomach acid to begin to turn. We worry they won't show up on time, or at all. And if they do show, they may take more than the allotted appointment time. They seem to enjoy creating disharmony within us and our office settings. They may doubt our intentions, and may not pay for the services rendered.

We may secretly wish that our schedules and patient logs were filled with those reliable, appreciative, trusting patients, but it is usually the patients that tend to drum up the drama, that teach us the most. They encourage our professional growth by challenging our knowledge and experience. They press us up against our personal limitations and require us to show more patience, ingenuity, integrity, and organization.

But if every patient we saw required this type of intense developmental growth from us, then we would shortly tire. Within the comfort growth cycle, there are certainly times for this intense development, but there are also times of quiet rejuvenation.

Think for a moment about how nature uses the comfort growth cycle to continue to develop and evolve. Each Spring, the challenge of growth is upon the world. Plants that have rested through Winter are now ready to bud, to deepen their root structures, to flower, to bear fruit, to sustain through the heat of the Summer, and then to release once again into the comfort of Autumn and Winter.

If nature was one continual growing season, how soon until the soil was depleted, how long until the temperatures become unbearable? Nature depends on periods of dormancy, where those challenging growful tasks are laid aside, and a stillness prevails that allows for rejuvenation. The soil restocks with minerals from decomposing organic matter. The earth cools, creating space for the warmth of a future growing season.

Taking this metaphor to our professional development, we see there is a great purpose in pushing ourselves, prioritizing our growth. Taking a risk and exposing ourselves to new information, new technology, new opportunities. These allow us to evolve. This expansive behavior is the lifeblood of our existence. We are creators, inventors, doers. The human mind and body seem pre-programmed with an innate desire to reach higher, run faster, metabolize more information. Our souls seem to speak to us of a journey of development and growth, and our bodies respond to that invitation. We resonate with that desire to accomplish, improve, and progress. This is our season of growth and development, our Spring and Summer.

There is also great purpose in allowing ourselves rest, peace of mind, acceptance, patience, and validation. This becomes our Autumn and Winter. We rest on a foundation of familiarity in these comfort cycles. We feel joy in our previous accomplishments and let them serve to encourage and embolden us to step toward the next necessary risk. We allow the progress and development we made during our last growing season to find a firm place within us. We update. We equalize. We prepare.

This comfort phase speaks of nurturance and validation. It feels safe in this part of the cycle. It is often tempting to stay here. It's understandable to desire this familiarity. Nature and human development, however, have a way of encouraging growth. Old trees that once sheltered and mentored the younger trees fall to the earth and open the canopy above to expose the younger trees to more challenges. The younger trees develop the strength to rise and take the place of the older ones.

It's worth considering how we are each uniquely being invited to grow, today, this week, this month. Our patients provide us regular opportunities to experience that need for growth. We are, at times, pressed up against our own limitations as we interact with challenging personalities and complicated clinical care. There is a feeling of dignity and nobility as we step toward those challenges with humility and integrity.

We may feel the discomfort of risking, of feeling inadequate and insufficient in the growth phase, but that is the springboard of development. When we rest for a moment in the comfort cycle we feel the gratitude and self-respect of a job well done.

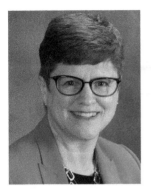

Colleen T. Fogarty MD, MSc, FAAFP, is the William Rocktaschel Professor and Chair of the Department of Family Medicine at the University of Rochester Department of Family Medicine. She earned her MD degree at the University of Connecticut School of Medicine in 1992. Dr. Fogarty is considered an expert in writing 55-word stories and using them as an educational tool for self-reflection. She has published many of these stories, poetry, and narrative essays in several journals.

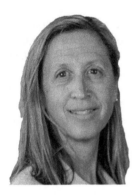

Amy Davis MD, MPH is a faculty physician at St. Mary's Family Medicine Residency and has been the medical director of the Western Colorado HIV Specialty Care Clinic since its inception in 2000. She attended medical school at SUNY Buffalo and completed residency at Maine Dartmouth Family Medicine Residency. Additionally, she enjoys trail running, skiing, fly fishing and travel.

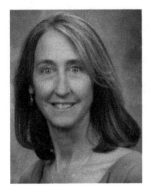

Lucy Graham PhD, MPH, RN, is the Director of Nursing Education Programs at Colorado Mesa University. She completed her doctorate in Nursing at the University of Colorado Anschutz Medical Campus in 2016 and maintains a clinical practice in a federally-funded clinic for people living with HIV in western Colorado. Outside of work she enjoys trail running, biking, skiing, reading, and traveling with family and friends.

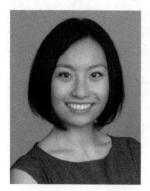

Alice Yuxi Lu is a student at the University of Massachusetts Medical School. She is currently in her fourth year of medical school and is applying to residencies to pursue her dream of becoming a pediatrician. Outside of school, she enjoys reading for pleasure, running, dancing, traveling, and photography.

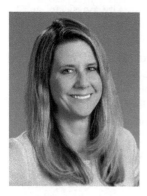

Jennifer Hodgson PhD, LMFT, is the Nancy W. Darden Distinguished Professor and Director of the Medical Family Therapy doctoral program at East Carolina University. She earned her doctorate in Human Development and Family Studies with a specialization in Marriage and Family Therapy from Iowa State University in 1997. Outside of work she enjoys spending time with her husband, Steve, and three children (Lauren, Ava Lynn, and Brennon).

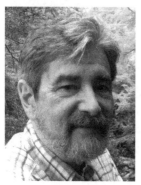

Mark P. Knudson MD, is Vice Chair in the Department of Family and Community Medicine of Wake Forest University in Winston-Salem, North Carolina. He completed his medical degree at University of Virginia, and his Family Medicine Residency and Fellowship at University of Missouri-Columbia. Outside of work he enjoys biking, hiking and spending time with his wife and 3 children.

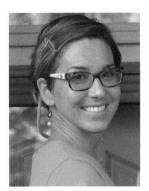

Kathryn Warren Hart DDS, is a pediatric dentist at Marillac Health in Grand Junction, CO. She completed a residency in pediatric dentistry at The Children's Hospital, Denver, CO in 2008 and an AEGD Residency at the VA Hospital in San Antonio, TX in 2004. She has taught dentistry students at CU and at Pacific Schools of Dentistry. She enjoys audiobooks, family and friends, and of course, flossing.

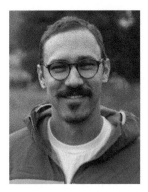

Justin H. McCarthy MD, is a faculty physician at St Mary's Family Medicine Residency. He received his Medical Doctorate from Creighton University where he also attended for his Bachelor of Arts in Medical Anthropology. Still a gosling of medicine, when he isn't boning up on medical knowledge he spends a great deal of time exploring desert trails by foot and bike, home brewing beer, succulent gardening, and trying to keep up with his wonderful wife.

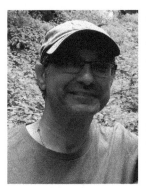

Arnold Goldberg MD, is the Assistant Residency Director of the Kent Family Medicine Residency in West Warwick, RI. He completed his Medical Degree from Rush Medical College in 981 and completed his residency in Family Medicine at St. Joseph Hospital/ Northwestern Family Medicine Program in 1984. He is a member of the AAFP, STFM and American Balint Society. He is a credentialed Balint Group Leader. Outside of work he loves to spend time with his wife and children and 5 grandchildren who all live nearby him.

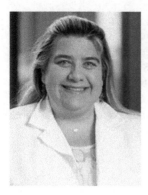

Jennifer Ayres PhD, ABPP is a board-certified, clinical psychologist from Austin. After 12 years in graduate medical education as the Director of Behavioral Health at the University of Texas Dell Medical School Family Medicine Residency Program, she took her current position as the Director of Psychology at the Rawson Saunders School and opened a private practice, Still River Counseling. In her free time, Jennifer enjoys traveling, writing, and having new adventures with her twin sons and their rescue dogs.

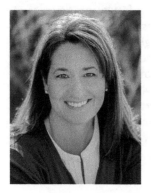

Juli Larsen BS, C-MI, is a meditation instructor in Grand Junction, CO. She completed her undergraduate work at Brigham Young University, majoring in Health Promotions. She enjoys philosophical conversations with her husband, discussing good books with her 5 children, and spending precious quiet time swimming and gardening.

Colleagues and Collaborators

Electronic supplementary material The online version of this chapter (https://doi.org/10.1007/978-3-030-46274-1_4) contains supplementary material, which is available to authorized users.

Her Reality

Colleen T. Fogarty

Tears of rage,
Overwhelming frustration–
"I love my work" she declares-
"I'm tired of leaving in tears at day's end
Teach me—I will learn—respect me."
Would that her peers could recognize her skills, her value—
She experiences discrimination, humiliation
Her perception is her reality
Her dedication, perseverance and skill
Devalued by racist discrimination.

Collaborative Partnerships and the Power of Connection

Amy Odom and Amy Romain

Amy O: It is Thursday evening. I furiously type my last few note attestations, determined to finish my computer work before I go home. It has been a long week on the inpatient service. I am physically and mentally exhausted. Finally, I close my laptop and quickly walk down the dark quiet hall where my academic office hides. The staff and residents have gone home. All the office doors are closed except Amy R's. I look in and mockingly ask, "What are you still doing here?" knowing I am guilty of the same trespass. She looks up and I see the distress in her eyes. She responds to me stating she is trying to write an email in a way that she won't regret, one that I know she probably should not send. I sit down to hear her story and send vibes of gratitude to my husband who by now has our kids fed and bathed. She goes on to tell me about an email she had received earlier in the day that put into question the years of work she dedicated to establish our integrated care practice. Her eyes welled with tears. Her words and posture carried the frustration of the struggle. In our safe space she confides, "It might be time to abandon this fight. It seems unwinnable." I glance over at a poster on her office wall office that reads, "Do the next right thing, one thing at a time, that will take you all the way home". She sees it too and files the email, deciding to come back to it on a later day.

Amy R: Amy O was right. I was exhausted and felt discouraged and devalued. For several years, I have led our practice transformation into integrated care. Others joined me along the way but I carried the torch for this cause. I knew giving up would jeopardize the model and worse, leave nothing to reflect my effort. That night, I was grateful to Amy O for meeting me in my distress. She could have just passed by my office and headed home, but she didn't. While she could not affect the change I needed at a system level, the power of her support and understanding kept me grounded and gave me the stamina to focus on doing the next right thing.

We came together several times for brief periods of work that day. In the morning, we met with our program director and shared our concerns for an intern's well-being. We discussed intervention strategies. We worried together about all of our interns and how hard the first month can be for them. We met over lunch to fine-tune our behavioral science curriculum schedule for the year. We cross-referenced our cal-

> The timing was perfect. We needed one another to validate each other's work. And so we began, behaviorist and physician, creating and presenting curriculum around family-oriented care.

endars, plans for vacations, and joked about the work we constantly create for ourselves because we are never satisfied with the way things have been done in the past! This snapshot of a day as collaborative partners is reflective of a relationship that has been ascending over the past 15 years.

Amy R: In the fall of 2002, I was the new, six hour per week behavioral scientist in our residency program. I was relieved to learn of the robust curriculum for psychopharmacology and communication skills, taught by physician faculty, but the remainder of the behavioral science curriculum would be up to me. It had been years since there had been a behavioral scientist on faculty and there were no resources or supports in place to guide me in my role. I was a bit at sea. The following year, the physicians who led the communications curriculum invited me to accompany them to the Forum for Behavioral Science in Family Medicine. I connected with people doing similar work and was encouraged by the generosity and collaboration among behavioral scientists and family doctors in this community.

Amy O: In 2002 I started residency in the same program as Amy R. I was mentored by physicians who were teachers of behavioral science. After I graduated, I accepted a faculty position in the residency program and soon thereafter completed a faculty development fellowship. This was a formative experience which helped me identify a deeper connection with the behavioral science field and focus my initial work around family-oriented curriculum development.

The timing was perfect. We needed one another to validate each other's work. And so we began, behaviorist and physician, creating and presenting curriculum around family-oriented care. As we grew together, we learned to trust each other, play on each others' strengths, and offer grace when things did not go as we had hoped.

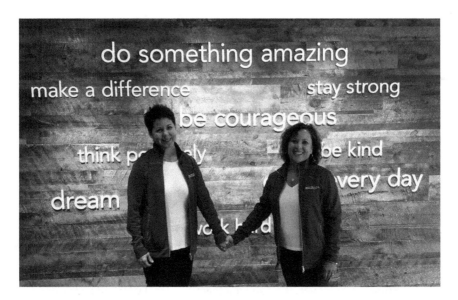

Amy O: Our first presentation together definitely required a little grace. As we stood at the reception desk checking into the hotel, we realized our handouts were missing. Amy R had been responsible for the handouts, but she left them in the taxi. Neither of us caught the taxi driver's name or his company. Our relaxing evening turned chaotic as we figured out expensive ways to recreate the handouts at the hotel. Fortunately, we had more ladders than chutes during this phase and our relationship was able to keep ascending.

Our growing connection promoted a desire to know more about each other. We felt safe enough to share our vulnerabilities and began to recognize the strengths each brought to the relationship. The energy generated through our collaboration fueled our work and resulted in creativity, innovation, courage, and outcomes that far exceeded what we could do alone.

Amy O: I vividly recall our first resident intervention together which was pivotal in building the trust needed for this stage of our relationship. This took place after teaching the first block of our new Intern Behavioral Medicine Rotation several years ago. It was clear to us that one intern was struggling. Though his medical knowledge was adequate, there was a great mismatch with his actions and the professional role he was supposed to be fulfilling. He did not see it, but everyone else could. Amy R and I identified a shared value; we both knew this needed to be addressed, even though it felt hard. We were invested in him as a person and as a physician. At the time, the culture of our program was to leave this sort of thing alone. Amy R and I were committed to doing the hard thing. In order to intervene, we had to recognize each other's strengths and trust that we would support each other. Amy R brought skills and experience to this task. I was intimidated, but carried the impact of being a physician. The result was a successful early intervention with someone who was grateful for the opportunity to reflect and grow.

As a result of our growing trust and connection, we began to identify with one another's priorities and values and eventually came to see them as our own. Now, when we sit across the table from each other during our weekly senior behavioral science teaching sessions, we perform a contemporary dance, alternating who takes the lead, improvising new steps, and ending in a final bow with hands joined. Our partnership has become so fluid, it is not always apparent who the physician is and who is the behavioral scientist.

Amy R: Recently, Amy O spoke on behalf of our practice as a panelist during a community conversation about integrated care. I watched and listened as she used the power of her physician voice to advocate for the implementation and expansion of behavioral health integration in our community. Despite being the integrated care champion in our program, I did not feel a need to be on the panel. I trusted her. What's important to me was important to her, because of our relationship. I knew her words and wisdom would make an impact because this was now our project.

Through the years, our collaborative relationship has grown from teaching partners on the subject of family to building and leading a 3-year behavioral science curriculum. We have presented over 30 times together at national conferences. We have tackled resident crises and led the way for earlier resident interventions. We have fought for practice transformation with integrated care and found creative ways to pursue this. We have grieved with each other when parents died or were given poor diagnoses and provided support when we each faced personal health concerns. We have processed the challenges and celebrated the joys as our families grow up and through the family life cycle. Our partnership has not always been this way. Indeed, this is hard to remember. We take for granted the ease with which we slip into each other's days and support each other's roles. The rewards we get from working collaboratively so far exceed the difficulties that we don't think twice about it.

Amy R: Like many others, our program has been through some tough challenges: program director turnovers, serious illnesses amongst our team, the spotlight of a national scandal. Amy O. and I leaned into the role of providing a holding environment for the people in our program. In times of distress, behavioral science faculty are often the open door, the shoulder, the glue. We show up and respond, no matter what is on our to-do list for the day. Yet, we should not do it alone. The weight of holding these things is diffused when the stress is shared and we are bolstered by resilience from our relationships.

The challenge for us now comes as we look forward. We have succeeded in creating a meaningful partnership that has spawned many successes. However, as our professional roles change and our trajectories shift there are more demands that compete for our time. A hard question remains - When will our collaboration end? We strive to make an impact in our program and our professional communities. Yet in the end, we do not really know what legacy we will leave. Perhaps, the greatest gift from our collaborative partnership is the joyous and enduring impact it has on our personal lives.

Adapting to Culture Change: Lessons from an Immigrant Child's Experience

Glenda Mutinda

"I'm so ecstatic!" That's exactly how I felt weeks before my family and I immigrated to the United States from Kenya. I could barely contain my excitement as I told my friends at school about the big move. Though we were no strangers to moving, as my family had done so several times while living in Kenya, this was by far the biggest move we had ever made. My recurring thought was, "I'm going to do EVERYTHING!" By the age of 10, I had already learned the importance of open-mindedness, optimistic curiosity, and a sense of adventure.

After we arrived in our new country, there were a lot of differences between my peers and me as well as my old environment and my new one. At times, I couldn't quite relate to everyone else; I didn't think their jokes were funny (and vice versa), and we had a hard time communicating because I spoke British English. I distinctly remember telling one of my new friends that I liked her spectacles. This simple compliment took almost 10 minutes to explain leaving both of us feeling frustrated.

Over time, however, my friends and I learned to laugh at our misunderstandings and to communicate better. I learned to explain why I spelled color with a "u" and wrote the date backward, and they learned to explain the cultural context of jokes so I could laugh, too. Such mutual learning allowed us to share our unique perspectives while maintaining our individuality. We learned to understand and appreciate each other's world views.

Due to my cultural and linguistic differences, there were still a lot of misunderstandings about my culture, my abilities, and me. My fourth-grade teacher, Mr. Fuller, became my champion in the school system. He was non-judgmental, objective, and curious to learn about me. He helped me fit in as much as he helped others recognize that I wasn't that different from them. One day, one of my classmates called me the "n" word and while I didn't know what it meant, I knew it wasn't a compliment. The first person I told was Mr. Fuller and upon learning what happened, he proceeded to address the issue with all my classmates. In the middle of class one day, he announced that we needed to have a serious conversation. He didn't "out me" as the person who'd had this issue, but he informed everyone that it was "simply not acceptable" to use derogatory language toward anyone in his classroom. The respect my classmates and I had for Mr. Fuller allowed for this message to be heard and accepted without challenge. That message helped me feel safe, supported, and like an equally valued member of the class.

> The complexities of my family's immigration journey from Kenya to the United States is very similar to my journey transitioning from traditional mental health to an integrated primary care setting.

The complexities of my family's immigration journey from Kenya to the United States is very similar to my journey transitioning from traditional mental health to an integrated primary care setting. Learning the language of integrated primary care was just as awkward as switching from British to American English. For example, I had to recognize that "MI" meant Motivational Interviewing for me and myocardial infarctions for my medical colleagues. I had to be flexible and open to experiencing a new system and culture to be an effective team member. Just like writing the date, I learned that while both methods of communication were valid, one method was better for each setting.

As I continued to collaborate with my medical colleagues, we learned how to better work as a team and I learned to balance my family therapy values, such as systemic thinking and family-oriented care with medical values of treating acute complaints. When a patient diagnosed with diabetes and depression came to the clinic, I stopped myself from assuming that attending to psychosocial needs isn't always important, if the treating provider chose to address diabetes first. Instead, I learned that there's a place, time, and purpose for practicing different skills and that same patient could be scheduled for a follow-up visit to discuss depression. My colleagues and I utilized each other's expertise when appropriate. For example, when a patient came to see me but was experiencing side effects from medication, I consulted with my physician colleagues and when their patients had biopsychosocial–spiritual stressors, they consulted me.

Though it doesn't happen often now, I sometimes have difficulties with belonging in the biomedical world. For those moments, I have continued interactions with other family therapists. Like Mr. Fuller, my supervisors and mentors have been instrumental in reinforcing the family therapist in me. Mentorship has been crucial to my ability to navigate the professional worlds I exist in. This relationship has allowed for my growth through modeling, conversations, building my professional networking, and on-going support.

It has been especially important for me to be an active agent for culture change through on-going, systemic engagement. As a young professional, using my voice to advocate for my services and field can feel intimidating, especially in a system that's built on hierarchies. I've learned to use my unique perspective to offer a different point of view in patient care, teaching, supervision, and developing and implementing policies. The beauty in being a new member of a system is the ability to see things through fresh eyes and use my voice to speak for change.

This process resembles that of my immigration experience. I found myself being an advocate for culture change for my parents as I often saw things differently than them. When they were concerned about me driving at age 15 years, I advocated for myself by offering a new perspective. I informed them that my driving would make everyone's lives much easier as I would be more independent. This meant I could drive my brother and me to school, I could run minor errands for them, and I could get a job as soon as I turned 16. With that argument, there was no way my parents could say "no." Similarly, I found myself being an advocate for culture change in integrated primary care, especially as related to how I work with physicians to treat patients with complex biopsychosocial–spiritual complaints. Some physicians would argue that addressing all presenting complaints would simply take too long. To address their concerns, I advocated for co-visits in which physicians could leave the visit appropriately after addressing biomedical concerns and get to the next patient. I would then finish the visit by addressing the psychosocial–spiritual concerns and plan a debrief with the physician at a more convenient time. Doing so would allow us to treat the patient's complaint in a patient-centric and timely manner with a method that did not interfere with the physician's workflow.

Sustaining culture change is as much a job for the champions in the system as it is for the professionals integrating into the system. The champions continue to use their power to keep integration going and new professionals can offer fresh ideas. Both are equally important. Any big change, whether immigrating to a new country or integrating into a medical system, means taking risks, functioning outside your comfort zone, and being part of a much bigger system that functions beautifully when filled with minds that think differently but working toward the same goals.

Reflections on a Personal and Professional Partnership

Michael Olson and A. Catalina Triana

Alone I go faster. Together we go further.

– African proverb

Act I: Initial Bonds and Shared Vision

Some individuals are fortunate to build lifelong friendships at work while others remain deeply connected at home without crossing the professional threshold. We are fortunate to have traversed both.

We met in training. Catalina had graduated from her family medicine residency program in Texas and was in a family systems medicine fellowship. Mike was a postdoc behavioral medicine fellow. Beyond a shared training location and commitment to similar clinical ideologies, we had very little in common.

Catalina, a 5' Colombian fireball, was raised as a free-wheeling, atheist liberal. Mike, a 6' 5" former college football player was raised in Utah as a member of the Church of Jesus Christ of Latter-day Saints. "An atheist and a Mormon walk into a bar..." sounds like the start of a bad joke rather than the beginning of a meaningful friendship. During the initial interview process for Mike's position, Catalina and her husband were asked to meet and greet Mike over dinner (not drinks, fortunately).

Within minutes of being seated, it was clear that this gentle giant and little firecracker would become great friends. As we shared our histories and vision for building integrated mental health teams in primary care, we identified common threads that united us; most importantly a shared value and commitment to improve healthcare. Mike sought to integrate mental health into medicine and Catalina strove to shape family medicine education to include mental health. Beyond the academic discussion, we also learned that evening how our personal and family histories shaped the ways we had come to relate to ourselves and others, further bringing our values into focus. The differences that could have divided us did not outweigh our common values and commitment to resident education.

> A central theme being that partnership works when there is a deep respect for one another and each person encourages change that will lead to personal and professional growth for themselves, the other, and the relationship.

As our training journey began we worked to support each other and grow as a physician–behaviorist duo. Beyond work, our personal lives began to intersect as our families began to share the joys and challenges of raising children.

Act II: Moving Apart, Growing Together

Catalina: After finishing fellowship, I returned with my family to our home in Colombia to fulfill training visa obligations. The departure was difficult for both Mike and me as we had built the beginnings of a training model and approach that would need to wait for two years to re-germinate. While in Colombia, I was able to find a new path supporting a new medical school in Bogota. A few years later, I was recruited back to Texas as a member of the residency faculty, partnering again with Mike and our team.

Mike: As Catalina left with her family to Colombia, I remained as a new member of the faculty. Maintaining continuity in our relationship during this separation was difficult. Our shared vision remained strong internally but there was limited collaboration. It became a time of personal development and growth for me. Catalina's return was a joyful reunion both professionally and personally.

These few years working from different institutions and in new roles provided unique growth opportunities for each of us. We learned to navigate different systems and struggle to implement our professional vision without the support of each other. This informed a new stage in our relationship as we again joined hands as faculty rather than trainees.

Our shared core values and being mindful of each other served us well as we rolled up our sleeves and got back to work. For the next several years, we found a new rhythm teaching, developing new curriculum and methodologies of teaching, caring for patients, and for each other. At the same time, our director was nearing retirement and the institutional system was changing.

Mike: Downward pressure from the school of medicine and department to increase billable faculty time put a value on clinical productivity above all else. The educational mission suffered and I no longer felt congruence with my core values. A meager salary, a growing family, high cost of living all combined for us to look for work elsewhere. It was a truly heart-wrenching decision, but ultimately we decided to move our family to Omaha, Nebraska and join other friends and colleagues at another university-based residency program. There, I found fertile institutional ground to support education, research, and integrated clinical training model pursuits.

Again, a separation of two friends and colleagues who desired to continue their work together. As we sat together on multiple occasions and discussed the challenges in the department at the time, there was compassion and positive regard and efforts to provide support moving forward. This time apart gave each of us another opportunity to develop our individual identities and talents as clinicians, educators, and scholars in partnership with new colleagues and peers.

Mike: With moving fatigue settling in, we settled into build a future in Omaha. Catalina's and my ability to maintain continuity and connection in our relationship during this separation improved. While the distance made this more difficult, we continued to have frequent contact, collaboration, and found ways to stay connected. It was a potent reminder that in order to maintain the direction and momentum of partnership there has to be intention and space to do so. When together, it seemed to flow so naturally; when apart, it often felt like swimming upstream.

Catalina: I continued to build my vision for residency education and championed the physician-behavioral scientist role, stepping into the Associate Program Director (APD) position with a program director who was a fierce advocate for integrated care, biopsychosocial medicine, and our team. I was offered the Behavioral Medicine Director position, but I insisted on a behaviorist leader and could not think of a better partner than Mike. In 2011, I reached back out to him to explore his potential interest in rejoining the faculty and to assume the director position.

Mike: After much thought and prayer, my wife and I revisited our Texas home and once again "tested the institutional waters" to see if there would be support necessary for another start. This time, negotiating from a different position for what was needed to be successful—professionally and personally. Now a family of seven, this decision was not taken lightly. The prospect, however, of meeting all of our needs drew us back once more and the journey resumed.

A new "dance" ensued. We worked to mindfully step, reconnect, rebuild, and renew our work together. An emerging complementarity of skills allowed us to help each other more effectively build toward the future. Examples of this include Mike working to support Catalina's goals of scholarship, publishing, and

disseminating her ideas and Catalina supporting Mike in his interests in motivational interviewing (MI) and becoming an MI trainer. A central theme being that
partnership works when there is a deep respect for one another and each person
encourages change that will lead to personal and professional growth for themselves, the other, and the relationship.

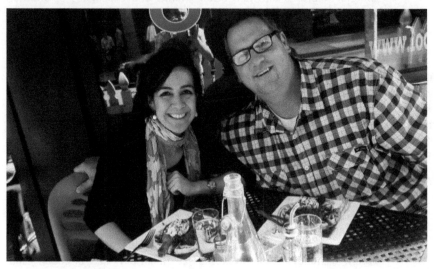

Another dimension that emerged as our partnership matured was the ability to
connect in a safe way and provide anchoring to each other during challenging
times. As anyone who works in complex systems knows, there are times when it is
necessary to "hold on to each other" to weather storms. These can be as
straightforward as threats to teaching time due to clinical productivity demands,
or more existential threats like whether the hospital and medical school will
continue after cataclysmic damage from flooding and natural disasters. Having a
strong base helped us to navigate these challenges together and fight to continue
our work.

We found teaching was more enjoyable when we were together than
apart. Residents shared with us that they learned not only about behavioral health
topics but also about interdisciplinary partnerships, collaboration, and mutual
respect when we worked together. We increasingly viewed our partnership as one
of our greatest assets and tools as scholars and educators.

These were productive and rewarding years, both of us growing professionally,
seemingly hitting our mid-career stride. APD, Director of Behavioral Medicine,
progressing academic rank advancement with tenure in sight, a clear focus and a
portfolio of successful work, publication, and presentations—all seemed to be
moving along as envisioned.

Act III: Supporting New Paths

Our time apart and together over the years had broadened the horizon and possibilities for the work we could do together and individually. We were both doing more consulting and training outside of our faculty jobs, including entrepreneurship and owning businesses. The eye of the storm passed in 2014 unfortunately and we again hit the institutional storm wall with clinic productivity and revenue generation straining education and time to teach residents. These, among other factors, left both of us open to new opportunities—although without clarity on what direction that would take.

Catalina: I was recruited to help build a family medicine residency program and clinic in the San Francisco Bay Area. A decision I now recognize as one of the hardest professional decisions I've made. Mike and I again parted ways as my family moved to the Pacific coast, taking the APD reigns and the task of building a new clinic and educational curriculum designed around integration of medical and behavioral health.

Mike: Not too long after Catalina took her new post in California, I was offered a position to join the faculty at a residency program in Colorado. The decision this time was compounded by leaving a program we had worked to build and older children at home. Again, after much reflection and prayer with my wife and family, we decided to pursue the opportunity to forge new partnerships with others committed to building integrated teams in primary care. This also brought us back to the mountain west and closer to aging parents and extended family.

While conflicted about yet another diverging path to our partnership, we both expressed a mutual desire and interest in the other's success, personal and professional development, and well-being. Many candid and difficult conversations ensued over the weeks and months that followed.

Epilogue

Before separating to our new residency programs, we committed to a plenary address on successful partnerships at a national conference. Preparing for this session required us to process our relationship at a difficult time, reflect on the journey and the challenges of moving in and out of each other's lives, and think carefully about what had made our work and relationship success.

Our presentation was a reflection on over 15 years of work together, deconstructing what we believed to be key elements of a successful partnership: sharing common goals and values, honoring the other's expertise, unconditional acceptance, compassion, and evocation of strengths that is based on mutual trust.

Mike: A message from a friend at the conference read: "What a tough decision for you both to make and how courageous for you both to make it. The grief between you and Catalina was palpable. Just wanted you to know you were in my thoughts." There was a sense of grief there, even if we hadn't fully acknowledged or embraced it at the time. Our focus was to stand together with our peers even as our paths had departed once again. Partnership has been hard work and has brought both joy and pain in the journey.

Now, several years later, we have been given yet another gift to reconnect, to process and heal a bit while writing this essay; to revisit the aspects of our partnership that have helped us over all these years and to again look to the future.

Physician Turns Patient

Mary Talen

The physician secretly shrouded the rush of terror attacks.
His stoic steel silence shielding him from eye-rolling judgments of peers.
Yet, charading as a cardiac attack, his panic was unmasked,
exposing him as a patient in need.
Oh, the twists when a physician turns patient-
He swallows the medicine of compassion to soothe sequestered pain.

Thriving

Alan Lorenz and Lisa Black

The following is a bit of "historical fiction," completely based on an actual case, but because the original psychologist was unavailable for authorship, her "inner voice" is supplied by Dr. Black. The final conversation is an actual conversation between Doctors Black and Lorenz.

Though well-liked, Eima was not a patient well-known to Alan. He did remember that she is a generally healthy 32-year-old graduate student from Iran. She called to have her rescue inhaler renewed, but since she had not been seen for over a year, she was scheduled for an appointment to review her asthma. She was scheduled for a time when Alan (her primary care physician) and Lisa (a psychologist) jointly saw all patients on Alan's schedule.

"Hi Eima, it's nice to see you again. I'd like to introduce you to Lisa, who is working with me today. She's a psychologist and on some days we see patients together—taking a whole person approach."

"Maybe we can start by talking about your asthma. I understand you need a new inhaler. How is your asthma going?"

"It's fine. I think I use my inhaler only a couple times a month at most. When I looked at the expiration, it was past expired. It really only flares up when I'm sick."

"Oh, that's great to hear and I'm happy to renew your prescription. Can I just take a quick listen ... Everything sounds normal ... I'm thinking Dr. Black might have some questions *::looks to Lisa and makes linking hand motions::* while I sit here at the computer, write up your note, and send in your prescription. *It always seems rude when I turn away and type, not making eye contact, but it always promotes conversation between the patient and Lisa—otherwise the patient answers her* *questions while looking at me ... and, it does help me get my note done, plus folding in their conversation makes my note better."*

"It's great to hear that your asthma is under control," Lisa affirms, "what's your sense of how that's come to be?"

"I'm from Iran and where I grew up, it was very dusty, and I think that had a lot to do with it. Also, both my brother and my mother had similar problems as children, and like me, pretty much outgrew it as an adult." *It's great that her asthma is under control but how can I be of help? Introduce diaphragmatic breathing to her?*

"Oh, that's wonderful. Do you do any special breathing techniques?"

"I just started doing yoga a few months ago, and there is a special breathing with that."

"Were you thinking that would help with your asthma?"

"No, not really, it's just something I always wanted to try, and I do it for the exercise and relaxation." *That is wonderful. I wonder what else I might help with.*

"I know graduate school is a stressful experience, believe me, I know ::laughter:: ... how are you doing in terms of managing your stress?"

"I believe I manage my stress well. I have a routine and get my work completed. I love my dissertation topic—gender roles in European theatre of the 19th century—and I look forward to learning more about it, and writing about what I do know, every day. My advisors are terrific and it's just so interesting to me!" *That is impressive. I still wonder if there is something she could improve.*

"Wow, that is an interesting topic! Even so, I know that writing a dissertation can really occupy your mind and sometimes affect your sleep. How are you sleeping?"

"I have a pretty solid routine, going to bed every night about 11 or 11:30, after talking to my husband, and get 7½ hours every night."

"Talking to your husband?" *Found it—relationship issues. I can help with that.*

"Yes, he is a research fellow at Harvard. That's part of the success of our relationship—we don't see each other that much! ::Laughter from all of us:: Seriously, he is very supportive. We talk or FaceTime every night and he comes back home to Rochester every other weekend or so. We both are very focused on our work and very productive during the week, and then, when we are together, we try to just be together. It works for us!" *Hmm, seems like she is really doing well. I can't be of much help. Maybe I can just join in her success and better identify factors that make her thrive.*

"It sounds like you are successfully meeting all the challenges of being in graduate school and having a quasi-long distance yet mindful relationship—in fact, I would say, you are thriving! Anything else you are doing or would like to do more of that would help you continue to thrive?"

"Hmmm … yes, that's so nice of you to notice and I am really happy with how things are going. Adding in yoga has been a nice addition. I certainly didn't need to do it, but it's made my life even better. It's been interesting for me to see how sometimes when I add in things that I want to do, even though it is extra time and energy, both of which are in short supply, it gives me energy and just creates this positive feedback loop. I guess along those lines, I also started auditing a class on gender roles in modern film. It relates to my dissertation, but a different media and a different time. I didn't really intend for it to be part of my dissertation work —I was just doing it out of interest and for fun—but it has introduced me to some new terms, and more importantly, maybe, introduced me to some new people. I might even get a job out of it! The gender studies department is looking for a new instructor in 1 1/2 years and here's hoping I will be all done by then!" *This is so great but I feel like I still need to add something to be of help. Make it worth her while for coming in.*

"You are truly an inspiration, and I applaud all your successes. The only thing I might add would be to learn some diaphragmatic breathing through biofeedback training. It might help further minimize the effect your asthma has on you."

"I have heard of that, and would be interested."

After the patient leaves, Alan and Lisa discuss the case.

"What a wonderful young woman," Lisa exclaims. "I am just disappointed I couldn't be of more help."

"I'm always happy to see people who are doing well, but yes, I don't know how much we really helped her."

"Isn't it weird though? We are almost disappointed that she didn't have any issues."

"Brilliant observation. As doctors we are taught to look for pathology, and when we don't find it, we almost feel like we didn't do a good job. This is such an important thing for us to know, and to teach our trainees. Looking for how our patients thrive both empowers the patients, and relieves us providers of that sense of disappointment when there is no pathology. Redefining helping to include a promotion of thriving brings a different type of fulfillment for all of us. And, joint appointments offer such a rich opportunity for this to occur."

"All true. We don't pay enough attention to the things our patients are doing right. When I hesitantly switched to focusing on the positives in her life she lit up and we learned so much more about her. Most importantly we learned some of her strengths. I think that helped build the relationships between us all. I also feel like if an issue were to ever come up with her I would lean toward using her strengths as a means to a solution instead of seeing them as just ancillary."

Lisa continues, "I'm also thinking about the differences between resilience and thriving. Resilience is the successful negotiation of challenges—the ability to overcome trauma, and other obstacles, both physical and mental. With thriving, the challenge is generated from within the self, not necessarily overcoming an obstacle. If we make it a point to ask positively focused questions like—What is going well in your life, what are you doing to challenge yourself further, and take it to the next level? This acknowledges, and maybe even promotes healthy growth. It offers a different vantage point of what healthy means for that particular individual. If in six months, Eima stopped yoga and didn't talk to her husband nightly, I normally wouldn't pay much attention to it. But, now, knowing that this is a part of her thriving way of life, we have a better understanding of when possible pathology might be forming, and how her strengths can be used as tools and protective factors."

"Totally agree. What an incredible tool we tend to ignore. And, I am so glad you were in the room for this one to help take us all to the next level. You make my job so much more interesting and enjoyable!"

I Am Lucky to Have Her

Christine Runyan

"Sara" entered the exam room as I imagined she might enter a courtroom under different circumstances—well dressed, walking with a confident stride in front of her husband, and fully prepared, clutching her stack of articles, consultant reports, and notes. Once in the exam room she sat in the first available seat, leaving the chair behind the exam table for her husband, seeming to indicate for all of us the relative importance of his opinion. As she tearfully described her uncertainty about whether to have surgery, she would occasionally flip to a page in her stack and re-read what she had already committed to memory, as if the answer might still be buried in there somewhere. Her PCP's attention was fully devoted to her as she spoke, moving away from the computer to avoid the inevitable impulse to start clicking through her chart.

I drew my attention to her husband "Bobby" as she spoke; although he was empty handed, his fear about her having surgery was clearly a heavy weight on him. He glanced up at me and we shared a moment of resonance in which I was empathizing with his fear of losing her, his fear of becoming a single parent, his fear of having to bear the burden of telling their son what happened to mommy. The terror of reliving the possibility of her dying left him unable to bear witness to her current suffering. In turn, this left her feeling alone and unsupported as she tried to decide the best course of action.

Five years ago, I met Sara and Bobby under dire circumstances in the hospital. Sara had been diagnosed with fatty liver disease very late in her pregnancy, which precipitated an emergency Cesarean, and left her critically ill after delivery. She and her husband of 20 years were unable to rejoice in their expanded family as she was fighting for her life. The care team suspected postpartum psychosis because she refused to see her healthy baby boy. Sara was anything but psychotic

—she was traumatized, fearful, she would fall in love and then have to say goodbye to her son, and felt unable to be maternal toward him as modern medicine worked around the clock just to keep her alive. Not seeing him was her defense. I spent time during the course of Sara's long hospital stay listening and talking with her and Bobby, as well as helping the inpatient team navigate their complex family relationships and competing opinions about recommended medical care.

> Her PCP demonstrated a refined ability to sit with the patient's suffering and distress, without rushing her, turning away or trying to prematurely fix.

Sara's full recovery took well over a year. She is currently enjoying motherhood to an active, gregarious boy with a full head of blond curls, deep blue eyes, and one of those smiles that is equal parts charming and mischievous. She is also slowly returning to work as a lawyer. I have stayed in touch with her through the years, primarily seeing her when stressful events or big decisions, such as whether to have another baby, are brewing. It was under these circumstances that I found myself in an exam room with her and Bobby again.

Sara contacted me when she began having acute GI distress that her PCP originally thought to be an ulcer and treated her based on this diagnosis. Ultimately, the GI pain was later revealed to be pancreatitis. Additional testing discovered distal damage to her pancreas, most likely caused by the treatments she received five years earlier that were necessary to save her life. Distraught about feeling sick for months, her mood suffered and anxiety and memories about her previous illness haunted her. Well-intended affirmations from friends and others about her weight loss brought her to tears rather than smiles, because it was severe pain, not willpower, which caused her weight loss. She sought second and third opinions including an expert consultation in which immediate surgery was highly recommended. Her efforts for clarity landed her, instead, in the undesirable position of conflicting opinions. On one hand, this very risky surgery might reduce her suffering and risk of cancer from a necrotic pancreas. On the other hand, the likelihood of her having cancer now was low and the surgery would also require a splenectomy. I listened and then asked how I could help. Her response: *"I need to talk with my doctor. He knows my history, he will listen to my concerns, he will be honest, and knows me."* Her PCP, the same PCP who asked me to go see her in the hospital five years ago, made an appointment with her and her husband outside of a regular clinic session, knowing it would be well over the 15 minute allotment of time. Sara asked me to join, mainly to observe the conversation and help her reflect on it afterwards.

Throughout the visit, I witnessed an incredible exchange filled with generous listening, medical information with a careful review of the data, a recognition and direct apology for his wrong diagnosis early in the course of these new symptoms, and a balanced reflection of the pros and cons of both action and inaction.

Her PCP demonstrated a refined ability to sit with the patient's suffering and distress, without rushing her, turning away or trying to prematurely fix. He acknowledged and reflected back her anger, fear, and most recently, acute pain and suffering. He shared a few moments of self-disclosure about his own medical issues and decision-making process. The conversation was difficult, but not rushed; it was intensely emotional and personal, but stayed on track without blaming other clinicians. Finally, he made a clear statement of unequivocal advice but acknowledged that, ultimately, the decision about surgery was still hers to make. It was a message that she might have heard before, but one that she could not fully receive until everything else had passed between them. At that moment, I saw Sara soften her grip on the stack of medical records, Bobby's shoulders finally relax, and I noticed my own release of air, held too tightly, in anticipation of his recommendation.

When he expressed gratitude for her trust in him and for wanting him to help her sort through the various test results and opinions, she seemed a little shocked. Shocked because through all of this, she could never imagine going through any of this without him. She wouldn't. She understood he is not perfect and did not expect that. What she knew to be true is how much he cares, how he gives her the generous gift of time when needed, and that he is completely honest, without an agenda … and that has always been what she—what any of us—needs most.

Walking back to my office, I understood completely why she could never imagine navigating this medical decision without him. In my role as an integrated primary care psychologist, it is a gift to be privy to such intimate and honest disclosures of fear, mistakes, compassion, and hope. I reflected to him my awe at his ability to listen to her words, while simultaneously tuning into her affect, as well as his thoughtful and balanced explanations of facts versus opinions. "*Sara is lucky to have you,*" I said. He paused before replying, "*You know, I am lucky to have her actually. She teaches me a lot.*"

The Kindness of Others

David Conway

I love Obstetrics.

Kindness helped me survive the difficult times.

My oldest child was born when I was a second-year nursing student. At the time, I had no idea where that birth would lead me, and I clearly remember the absolute terror and beauty of it…bringing a life into this world that was part me, helping my wife survive a long labor in a hospital that did not yet offer epidurals, surviving my growing doubts and fears over three hours of pushing, while overhearing a nurse whisper to the midwife multiple times, "The heartbeat is only 70." At the time, I didn't know how to interpret this information, but I knew that whispering was bad. It was the midwife who saw my fear and reached out to give me a hug and reassure me that everything was really okay.

Only a week later, I started my maternity nursing rotation. Having just experienced labor and delivery up close with my wife, I started with more confidence than any of my peers, but never considered working as a Maternity Nurse—whoever heard of a male L&D nurse, anyway? And they had never had a male nurse before.

It took long months to earn the staff's trust and confidence. There were days in the beginning when my skills were rudimentary at best, when my clinical decisions were questioned, and when I was asked to do orderly jobs. Over time, I won over the confidence and friendship of the staff there and garnered the support I needed to apply to medical school.

One thing for which medical school cannot fully prepare future physicians is the reality of bad outcomes, and how to survive them.

There is an emotional journey that physicians go through alongside their patients when they experience loss. For me, the stress of managing terrifying labors that sometimes result in poor outcomes took a toll. To survive, I learned to accept the kindness of others.

One experience stands out in my memory. After residency, I practiced at a small rural hospital, a long 2½-hour drive to any tertiary center. A patient had switched to my practice at 26 weeks in her second pregnancy, after she had developed a chronic abruption. After intensive antenatal surveillance for the remainder of her pregnancy, she presented to the hospital full-term, in labor, and the nurses could not find a heartbeat. I was filled with trepidation as I searched for but was unable to find a fetal heartbeat.

> I stumbled out of the labor room in tears, wandering blindly down the hallway toward my call room. Margaret, a 60-year-old housekeeper, came seemingly out of nowhere and embraced me. She patted my back as her deep smooth voice repeated, *"Everything will be alright. It's okay. You did the best you could."*

When a bedside ultrasound confirmed a stillbirth my devastation and despair were overwhelming. Despite having had similar experiences during residency, I was so overcome, I could hardly get words out. This was the first time that I had cared for a patient with a stillbirth who had chosen me to guide her safely through pregnancy. My hands shook as I took hers in mine; my voice broke, and I barely choked out how sorry I was, that I was not sure why this had happened.

I stumbled out of the labor room in tears, wandering blindly down the hallway toward my call room. Margaret, a 60-year-old housekeeper, came seemingly out of nowhere and embraced me. She patted my back as her deep smooth voice repeated, *"Everything will be alright. It's okay. You did the best you could."*

As simple and empty as those words seemed in the moment, they somehow sustained me, somehow reassured me that I had the knowledge and skills to help this grief-stricken mother survive the next few hours, days, and weeks. That experience taught me that comfort and reassurance can come from the most unexpected places. In that moment, Margaret was as pivotal to my career as any previous experience.

Years later, while working at a family medicine residency, I was called in the early morning after neither the nurses, the on-call resident, nor the family medicine attending could find a heartbeat for a laboring patient.

"Dr. Conway is our OB/GYN expert," they told her. "He is great with ultrasound, and he'll be able to find the heartbeat." My heart pounded with the hope that I could live up to their promise, but my fears were realized when I, too, could not find a heartbeat.

"Your baby has died," I told her, trying to model for the resident physician how to embody presence and calm while delivering devastating news to a patient I was meeting for the first time. I struggled to hold back tears as I told her, "I don't know why this happened. I am so sorry for your loss."

Her response gutted me. She was inconsolable, and she literally screamed for twenty minutes straight. I sat with her, holding her hand. I whispered to her over and over that there was nothing that she had done to cause this, nothing that she could have done to prevent it, that I would stay with her, I would help her through her labor. Any pretense of fighting back tears disappeared; we were all sobbing.

I later debriefed with the first-year resident, who happened to be in the midst of her second trimester at the time. "I'll never do obstetrics," she told me, "I could never do what you just had to do." We talked about the physician tradition of emotional compartmentilization.

It has allowed me to step outside of my own emotions, in a sense, and stay in the moment to care for a devastated patient; it permitted me to somehow set aside my own devastation and be the physician the patient needed me to be. But, it comes with a cost over time.

Years later, on the verge of retirement, my oldest daughter, whose birth had pulled me into obstetrics 34 years earlier, found a lump in her breast. When I called a breast surgeon colleague at the hospital where I worked to arrange an appointment, I heard my own voice, strangled and cracking. I paused, took a deep breath, and stepped outside of myself to relay the relevant clinical and logistical information. After accompanying her to a mammogram, ultrasound, and consult with the surgeon, I numbly listened to the terrifying results that I had often delivered to patients in my own role as a physician: My daughter had Stage 3 breast cancer.

The world closed in around me as we discussed the likely diagnosis and plan. And, just like I had done throughout my medical career, when the world seemed to be going to hell all around me, I thought I knew how to keep on task focusing on what needed to happen next, medically. That ability allowed me to keep at bay the sheer terror that my first born had a life-threatening cancer and might be taken from me, and there was nothing that I could do to stop that. It allowed me to focus on helping her survive, but didn't stop the tears that came at seemingly random times.

Just as I had in the past, I found comfort from an unexpected place. After the diagnosis, my daughter contemplated her impending hair loss with chemotherapy. Several family members, friends, and I volunteered to shave *our* heads in empathy and solidarity. My barber was happy to oblige, using clippers to get my hair as short as possible so that I could shave my head at home. Seeing this supportive group become voluntarily bald, my daughter decided to do the same to avoid the gradual patchy loss of hair. She also went to my barber, who cut her hair down to stubble. Later, while I was shaving off the last of her stubble, she told me that he had not charged her for the haircut. This simple gesture of generosity just stunned me.

Months later, after both of us let our hair grow back in, I visited him again. Tears welled up in my eyes and I could hardly get the words out to express my gratitude. What must seem to others to be such a simple act of kindness had, again, just overwhelmed me.

Thankfully, my daughter is now a 5+ year survivor, with two toddlers; an added joy to my retirement! As I look back over my career I have learned and embraced the importance of sharing the value of kindness with residents—the kindness that I received as both a husband and then a father of a patient; the kindness that I have received from patients throughout my career; and the kindness that I have tried to bestow on patients. Kindness has a place in everyone's heart, and such a simple thing can help someone survive.

Music and Stories

Sarah Gerrish

When I listen to Ladysmith Black Mambazo, the stories that brought me to medicine flood my memory. Seventeen years ago, I spent a year in Malawi with Beata, my Polish roommate who spoke minimal English. We had no phone, radio, TV, or a flush toilet. I can still feel the sticky heat, taste the creamy custard apple fruit, hear the village singing behind the church, and see the colorful batiks wave among the friendly village smiles.

The memories are clear like no time has passed. I worked in the village dispensary, which functioned like an urgent care and had an adjoining one room maternity ward with four beds. Two weeks into my volunteer "training," I watched a midwife deliver two women simultaneously. The midwife turned to me in her white starched uniform and asked me to deliver the other baby. I was just "observing." "You must! Now!" she said while pointing at my hands. I had the last clean pair of rewashed latex gloves in the entire dispensary. Too many women had delivered that day and the midwife had not rewashed enough latex gloves.

I remember walking around the surrounding villages with Beata. One day, we found an emaciated 18-month-old boy with a terribly gangrenous leg and trouble ambulating. "No money for medicine," his mother said. She had neither soap nor clean cloth for bandages. Her son had burned his leg from boiling porridge several weeks ago. "We will help," I said in my poor Chichewa. We returned to her small mud-walled thatched roof hut every day to clean his wound and change his dressings. After a month, it healed, and he could walk normally again. Three months later, when the corn was being harvested, that mother came to us with a bucket of corn. "Thank you," she said and walked away. That amount of corn could have fed her family for a week.

In that village, wealth meant something entirely different. The Malawians lived meaningful, contended lives, stripped of possessions and basic needs in a culture rich in laughter and music. I felt the guilt of my privilege, gluttony, greed, and education. Despite all this, nothing felt so right. I made the decision. I want to be a doctor.

It all seemed worth it when I was an idealistic, naive, passionate, and an unattached 20-something. But seven years into medical training, as a second-year family medicine resident, married, and with a new baby, my inspiration had faded like the batiks on my wall. My passion was slowly being stripped from me with the hours upon hours that I spent training in the hospital and studying for tests while ignoring my friends, family, and my own health. What had I accomplished except complete checklists, requirements, professional metrics, be on time for rounds after pre-rounding at 5 am, do presentations, and be there for continuity deliveries? I couldn't even fill out the 9-month Ages and Stages form of my own son because he was perpetually in daycare. At that moment, I felt forced to choose between being a good parent and spouse, which made me appear like a disengaged doctor. Or I choose to be like one of my family medicine heroes and never see my family. I knew it was not that simple. But on the bad days, it seemed like I lost with every choice. My mind ruminated with the question: *Was the price I paid for this medical career worth the sacrifice?* The emotional, physical, and mental exhaustion was soul emptying.

My residency clinic was central in refugee medical care as it was located in a designated refugee relocation city. Nearing the end of residency, an Iraqi woman was brought in by her husband for weakness and fatigue. My own mental fatigue was drowned by the barriers that consumed this first 20-min new patient clinic visit. *Where would I even begin? How would we overcome the limits of language, mental illness stigma, discussing trauma, relocation stress and cultural isolation? How would we negotiate the financial and political roadblocks in this medically rich country?*

Then I remembered the music, my African neighbors had almost no material possessions. They possessed something richer, stories told in their music. Then, I remembered the stories of my medical beginning. People were dying of cholera because there was no access to medicine and clean water. Drought was causing neighbors to kill each other for food. USAID was being sold at the market. Boiled mice on a stick and flying fried termites were delicacies. My hats were pulled apart by the village women while they taught me to knit. These stories returned my heart, hope, and fire that was almost stolen through the rigor of medical training and demanding priorities of life.

This Iraqi woman had a story to tell me and that was where we started. Over many clinic visits, she described a life in Iraq where she loved to cook and sing. Her family was lucky to escape the violence. She felt grateful that her family was together in a new safe country. But now she felt no desire to sing. We attempted to discuss mental illness and what that meant in her language and culture. I slowly tried to understand the cultural and political climate of Iraq. Over the visits, the desperation and fatigue would fade from her face and she slowly regained some daily functioning.

Now when I listen to Ladysmith Black Mambazo, the stories find their rhythm in my life and remind me of the power of stories in my life and the lives of my patients.

This is the story of how we begin to remember
This is the powerful pulsing of love in the vein
After the dream of falling and calling your name out
These are the roots of rhythm
And the roots of rhythm remain
– Paul Simon, Under African Skies.

Unsiloing the Mystery

Angela L. Lamson

It was a wintery day in 1998, and there I sat at the end of a very long table, what in most workplaces would resemble a board room. The sixth floor, the inpatient behavioral health unit, was eerily quiet for the adult wing but particularly unusual that day on the adolescent side of the unit.

As a therapist in training, the daily rounds in this small hospital kept me on the edge of my seat. This morning I decided to sit in the middle of this never-ending table. Usually I felt much more comfortable in this room; it was where I met with families as part of a youth's treatment or discharge planning.

I caught myself listening to the way I held my breath as people took their seats. I glanced around the table with eyes wide open as one provider after another took the seat that only he or she typically claimed.

The psychiatric nurse to my right, who had been with the hospital almost as long as I had been alive took the seat next to me and threw me a half smile. Then sat the social worker who seemed to always be at the top of her game. I knew she would not sit long, because she was the first to ensure that the adolescents attended school during the day on the unit, and that both adolescents and adults had specified referral plans upon discharge.

Then there was the financial administrator, who I knew I would not fully appreciate until later in my career. Yesterday, I could hear her battling with an insurer, getting clearance for every treatment that a patient needed. Today's discussion would be tricky, as our newest patient had no insurance at all. I could see frustration already flushed across her face.

At the head of the table, the most intimidating seat of all, was the psychiatrist. That seat was *always* reserved for the psychiatrist. The psychiatrists (which in any meeting) started with either the adolescent psychiatrist or adult psychiatrist based on their availability and the patients we were discussing. Both psychiatrists were so well respected in the community. I was grateful we started this morning's review with the adult psychiatrist. I had shared many great collaborative conversations with him this week about the patients on the unit and their families.

One by one, we went around the table and shared the previous day's experiences that we had with patients. I recalled an adult male who somehow walked into the hospital with a blood alcohol level that would have ended the life of most people and then described an adult woman who experienced her depression as so deep that she could not remember the last time she experienced light from outside her home. There were other adult patients who received more attention from the social worker or financial administrator at the table.

As is the case with most patients who receive acute care in hospitals, I do not know what became of that young woman. I do know that her life story influenced me greatly and gave me the voice to advocate for family-oriented care on behalf of others like her, with colleagues who could help to make a difference.

Then it was time to discuss the adolescents. The psychiatrists passed one another at the door and the temperature of the room seemed to drop 10°. Why does that narrative always spin inside me when I meet with this psychiatrist? I could feel the messages of my imposter phenomenon take over as he took his seat.

A young woman, just barely 16, was described by most in the room as experiencing schizophrenic behaviors. No family came to see her yesterday. While I knew I was the one at the table with the least years of experience in treating severe mental health diagnoses, there were at least a few items I thought I could contribute. There were several things I wanted to say about larger systems experiences, but today I would say just two things.

"Excuse me", I said, "I realize that her toxicology report has not been sent to us yet. I also realize that we do not have much history on her care beyond what we have experienced since her arrival into the unit." The nurse, who typically could unlock the story of any patient's emotional vault, spoke up "she's not talking to anyone." The social worker concurred. I shared with them that the young woman let me talk with her this morning at length. I could feel the nurse and social worker lean in toward me and I was not sure if I should feel honored or anxious about their body posture.

"I think what we are witnessing is withdrawal from methamphetamine use." All eyes were on me as I unfolded what this young woman had shared with me. It was deep and dark and worth nurturing as she had been emancipated and thrown to the evils of the world. The narratives from each member around the table began to shift and everyone went into overdrive to find out how to assist this young woman from a life that would have otherwise ended too soon. My senses took over as I could hear each provider's pen taking notes of a professional action plan based on his or her experience and expertise.

Then, it was like my imposter phenomenon decided to put on a superhero cape for the morning. Words started rolling out of my mouth faster than I could stop them. "I just want to tell you what I have witnessed since joining this group of providers. I feel like we function as silos, a co-located bundle of experts that rarely act as an integrated team. Look at us today, this young woman was individually interviewed by at least four mental health providers, representing at least four mental health disciplines, at four separate times during the first 12 hours of her stay. We were cooperative, but rarely collaborative."

It was about now that my stomach had caught up with my mouth and I realized I should really stop talking.

The psychiatrist leaned in. "Go on."

"Rather than sharing a unified assessment that would have allowed all four disciplines at this table to maximize care with the patient; a patient's story often grows less and less detailed and more and more exhausted or frustrated as he or she shares and reshares their reason for admission. This great team can co-exist (while staying safe within our discipline) with very little impetus to collaborate or integrate care in treatment with one another."

I knew that my time at the hospital would soon be coming to an end as I approached graduation from my program, but leaving that room that morning felt like I had succeeded in overcoming something perhaps just as important as passing my dissertation defense. I met eye to eye with my imposter phenomenon and in the midst of it all, strengthened my relationship with this incredible team of providers. I cannot say I ever witnessed fully integrated care during the rest of my time on the unit, but collaboration increased and duplication of assessments was reduced.

As is the case with most patients who receive acute care in hospitals, I do not know what became of that young woman. I do know that her life story influenced me greatly and gave me the voice to advocate for family-oriented care on behalf of others like her, with colleagues who could help to make a difference. Through family-oriented care (however family is defined by the patient) health and illness can be navigated together rather than in isolation.

While fully integrated care may not be possible in every healthcare context, I have heard from countless patients and providers how invaluable integrated care can be and I have witnessed the research that supports the importance of collaborative care rather than treatment in isolation. So, I thank that young 16-year-old, whereever she may be now… that through her sacrifice and story came a provider who has spent her career advocating for families at the center of all healthcare.

Introversion in Team-Based Care

Jackie Williams-Reade

I park and walk into the clinic, through the empty waiting room, and into the front office on my way to my desk. I nod to Shari, one of the office coordinators, and say "Good morning." Shari and I are both introverts. We may not say a lot to each other, but we know we like each other as we exchange knowing looks and smiles in the midst of the busy clinic culture.

I walk past Steve, another office coordinator, and immediately feel some pressure to belt out a loud hello. This is how Steve likes to talk – loudly and emphatically. This kind of interaction often drains me, though sometimes after being well-rested I can fully engage and enjoy it. Currently, though, it's 7:30 a.m. and I can't summon up this level of performative energy right now. I say "Hi, Steve" with as much volume as I can muster in the moment, but know that this kind of greeting may not register with him.

I say hello to Denise, the third office coordinator, and know she will only give a mutter in response. Perhaps Denise is a fellow introvert, but I'm always a little perplexed why she responds in this manner. She is always engaged in business matters, and I respect that as deep focus is a common introvert trait. However, her lack of a simple hello makes me feel like she may not like me. I take note that this is how others likely feel when I give them my favorite introvert greeting of being quiet and not interrupting.

I head to fill up my water bottle in the break room. I'm relieved when I see the room is empty as unexpected interactions can really drain me. My introverted brain takes longer to think of things to say. Even if I'm asked a simple question like "how was your weekend?" and I haven't thought it through, I'm liable to sputter something incoherent and awkward. Gratefully, I don't have to navigate that conversation yet and I am glad for a bit of brain rest in this moment.

I grab the patient check-in sheets and review their notes on the computer. Dr. Harley's patients are here first, and I walk down the hallway to say hello to him. Dr. Harley and I get along well, much to the surprise of others in the clinic. Many say he is cold, distant, and intimidating. I can see through these characteristics, though, as they are used to describe my behavior as well when I am simply being quiet. You just have to find the right conversation and Dr. Harley brightens up, just like any introvert. We tend to talk about places in Montana as he loves the state and I am from there. We also swap stories about our days in Baltimore and at Johns Hopkins. Dr. Harley gives me many opportunities to work with his patients and often tells them how important my work is to their overall health. Working with him is easy for me while others in the clinic tend to leave him alone. It's nice to work in our small team in the mornings—a perfect introvert pair we are.

> I step into the next room and catch the elderly patient and her adult daughter by surprise. They know I am not their doctor and are confused as to why I am in their room. This unexpected reaction makes me nervous and the classic introvert lag time between my thinking about what I want to say and saying it occurs as they stare at me bewildered.

I walk into the first patient's room and convey an energetic greeting and introduction. It's a bit of a stretch for me to do this as my introversion can make me prone to approach others with some tentativeness, waiting for them to engage before I do. But I know a good greeting helps patients feel more at ease with me and gets me into the deeper interactions I crave as an introvert. My first patient is very open once I asked her a few warm-up questions and to tell me about the stress of living with an adolescent teen. I weave in ideas about this being related to her high blood pressure and we discuss ways to manage it all. It's an easy dialogue and I leave her room feeling good.

I step into the next room and catch the elderly patient and her adult daughter by surprise. They know I am not their doctor and are confused as to why I am in their room. This unexpected reaction makes me nervous and the classic introvert lag time between my thinking about what I want to say and saying it occurs as they stare at me bewildered.

In an ideal world, I could think through what I want to say which allows me to be clearer, but there is not enough time for me to think in this moment. Speaking clearly and thoughtfully is actually one of my greatest skills. However, when put on the spot (which happens constantly in team-based care), I often fumble my way through as I grasp for words. In this moment, I can tell I am losing the patient's and family members' confidence. I finally find the words I have been searching for and get them talking about their primary concerns. I exit, not feeling great about the encounter and taking a bit of a hit in my energy level from the interaction.

I run into one of the other behavioral health providers on my way back to my desk and we have a quick check-in about our weekends and how our morning is going. She is also an introvert, although she comes across as more bubbly and talkative than I do. Her weekends always include plenty of downtime like mine, and we bond over our need to get away from the clatter of the clinic at lunch time.

Eating together at lunch time is very important at this clinic. While I would prefer to eat on my own to help replenish my energy after a busy, conversation-filled morning, I make a point to eat in the lunch room a few times a week. On other days, I will run an errand or go find a quiet place to sit. When I return from my solo lunches, I'm consistently asked about my whereabouts over lunch. I find this so endearing that my colleagues miss my presence. Yet it is also peculiar to me that my absence is noted, because when I do eat lunch with everyone, I find I can hardly get a word in edge-wise. I require a lot of space to jump into a conversation —ideally about three seconds after one person stops talking is when I feel comfortable speaking without interrupting. These pauses are rare in a medical clinic, so I constantly work on feeling ok "interrupting" people, otherwise I will never get the chance to speak.

The extra work I do to fit into the extroverted culture is likely not recognized by many of my patients or colleagues. Despite these challenges, working as a part of team-based care is worthwhile to me as it is full of moments of deep connection and meaning with both patients and colleagues. My main contributions are valuable, though often quiet.

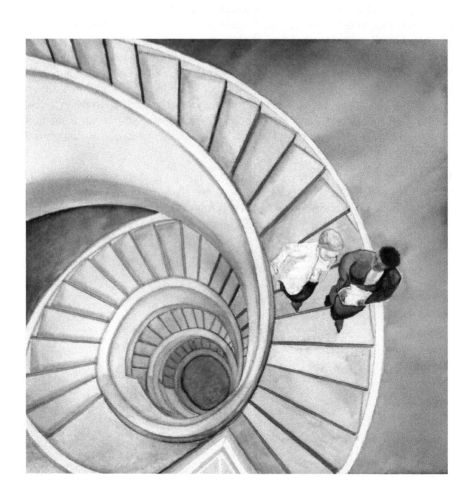

Reflection on Colleagues and Collaborators: Collaborative Curiosity

Juli Larsen

A twisted ladder
The unfurling fern
Threads on a common screw
A nautilus shell
A spiraling staircase

These are all examples of what we call a double helix. We are more familiar with a double helix when we speak in terms of DNA; but a double helix, considered art to many, has become a symbolic representation of upward growth, a collaborative alliance between two separate backbones, spiraling around a common purpose, joined together by values and shared experiences. Ultimately, the structure is organized in an effort to achieve both strength and a destination.

Workplace collaboration can also be modeled as a double helix, providing us a catalyst for the personal and professional development we yearn for. As a "backbone" in our workplace, we provide one of the necessary structural supports that will form the double helix. We spiral upward with our capabilities, goals, and experience. We bring our best, most prepared self. We do the work to develop our own unique individual identities, but if left on our own, we lack the structural stability to move upward under pressure. Collaborating with others, or forming a double helix, allows us to gain strength and support for a mutual purpose.

Collaboration starts with self-confrontation, an examination of our own backbones. We may ask ourselves: What is it like to work with me? What do I do that makes it hard to collaborate with me?

As we reflect on how we engage in collaborative relationships, we begin to see how we operate within the framing of a double helix. How are we in relation to the other partnered backbone? Are we overbearing, submissive, absent? Do we shrink from our personal responsibility, fearful of the risk and exposure that comes from fully participating? Do we micromanage others, getting a subtle sense of superiority from our inflated sense of self? How can we challenge our development in order to become a more collaborative partner? This process of self-definition encourages us to develop our own collaborative backbones first.

As we begin to strengthen our own backbone, we become better suited to the work of collaboration. That work at times can be uncomfortable, anxiety provoking. When we bring a more developed self, we are better able to tolerate the discomfort that collaboration at times invites. Instead of reacting to someone's feedback with a critical energy, we can explore together, what they are offering. Instead of our unconscious inviting us to feel threatened by someone's wisdom or input, we can experience more gratitude for their contributions. Instead of repeatedly trying to rescue someone, we can stay anchored to our shared goal and offer our genuine belief that they are capable of the task at hand. We can maintain clarity around the beauty of a common goal—a goal that we are equally invested in achieving.

Collaboration invites us to experience the tension of belonging to ourselves while we also belong to the group. It is not easy to lay claim to our own ideas and feelings, while cultivating space for different ideas or feelings. This struggle is often exhibited as defiance, the desire to conquer, or compliance, the desire to defer. Perhaps both of these dynamics, have at their root, a desperation to be right and a low tolerance for being wrong. The defiant gives no room for variation from their view, feeling a strong opinion will demonstrate how they are right. The compliant gives no counter view to consider, preferring instead to ride the coattails of someone else, enjoying feeling right if the idea is successful and feeling right if the idea isn't successful, because after all, it wasn't their idea. Collaboration is neither defiance nor compliance, but rather collaboration exists as a space set aside to explore differing ideas and thoughts, without the initial judgement of right or wrong. In this process of exploration, we are invited to belong to ourselves and the group. By voicing our thoughts and sharing our experiences, we belong to ourselves. By exploring other's ideas, we belong to the group.

Curiosity is the catalyst that allows us collaborative movement. Without curiosity, we can become rigid in our own views, somewhat protective of our own thinking and efforts, and at times this invites a defiant behavior. On the other side of the collaboration spectrum, without curiosity we may become overly nervous to expose our thinking, our questioning, thus we are invited into compliant behavior. As we nurture curiosity, we help create the collaborative space necessary for exploration. Curiosity becomes a way to move away from compliant or defiant behaviors.

Mario Testino, a world famous fashion photographer, has said:

My favorite words are possibilities, opportunities, and curiosity. I think if you are curious, you create opportunities, and then if you open the doors, you create possibilities.

Workplace collaboration spirals up on the platform of curiosity, creating the next opportunity, inserting the next step on the staircase, the next rung on the ladder, making the impossible, possible.

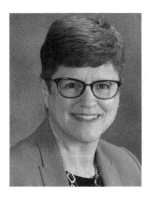

Colleen T. Fogarty MD, MSc, FAAFP, is the William Rocktaschel Professor and Chair of the Department of Family Medicine at the University of Rochester Department of Family Medicine. She earned her MD degree at the University of Connecticut School of Medicine in 1992. Dr. Fogarty is considered an expert in writing 55-word stories and using them as an educational tool for self-reflection. She has published many of these stories, poetry, and narrative essays in several journals.

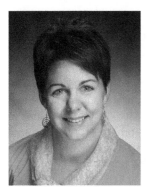

Amy Odom DO, is an Associate Program Director at the Sparrow/Michigan State University Family Medicine Residency Program in Lansing, Michigan. She completed her doctor of osteopathy at the Ohio University Heritage College of Osteopathic Medicine in 2002. She has published poetry and narratives in the journals Family Medicine, Family Systems and Health and the online site Pulse. Outside of work she finds joy in reading, gardening, and spending time at Lake Michigan with her family.

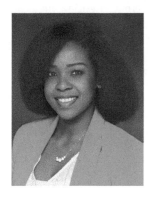

Glenda Mutinda PhD, LMFT, serves as the Director of Interprofessional Well-being at JPS Health Network. Dr. Mutinda holds a doctoral degree in Medical Family Therapy from East Carolina University and completed advanced fellowship training in behavioral health immersed in medical residency training programs. Her research interests include well-being of learners, diversity and health equity, and integration of behavioral medicine in healthcare.

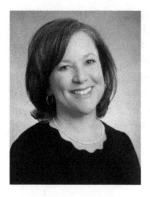

Amy Romain LMSW, ACSW, is the Director of Behavioral Medicine in the Sparrow/Michigan State University Family Medicine Residency Program in Lansing, MI. She completed her Master of Social Work degree at Michigan State University in 1995. She has published on the topics of physician well-being, interprofessional collaboration, behavioral science curriculum and the care of vulnerable populations. Outside of work she enjoys gardening, the arts, and spending time at the lake with family and friends.

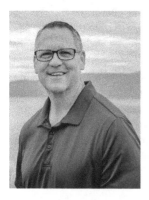

Michael Olson PhD, LMFT, is Director of Behavioral Medicine Education at the St. Mary's Family Medicine Residency program in Grand Junction, Colorado. He completed a doctorate in Marriage and Family Therapy at Kansas State University in 2001 followed by a post-doctoral fellowship in Behavioral Medicine from the University of Texas Medical Branch. Outside of work, he enjoys spending time with his wife and children, composing music, art, and all the outdoor activities life in the mountains offers.

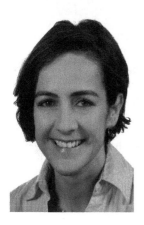

A. Catalina Triana MD, is a Family Physician, medical educator, and behaviorialist practicing in the Bay Area in California. She codirects the UCSF Northern California Faculty Development Fellowship. Her passion is to support people's growth and well-being.

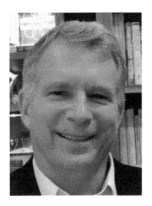

Alan Lorenz MD, is Clinical Associate Professor of Family Medicine and of Psychiatry at the University of Rochester. He completed residency in Family Medicine and Fellowship in Family Systems at the University of Rochester in 1991. He co-authored Models of Collaboration and Family-Oriented Primary Care. Outside of work he enjoys a wide variety of sporting activities, travel, and writing.

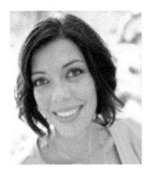

Lisa Black PsyD, is the Lead Therapist for Biofeedback and Neurofeedback Services at UCSD Family and Preventive Medicine Division, Collaborative Care. She has completed a doctorate in Clinical Psychology at Alliant International University, San Diego in 2016. She has been actively involved in improving behavioral health collaboration within her own clinic and through research studies. Outside of work she enjoys gardening and spending time outdoors.

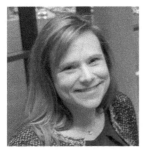

Christine Runyan PhD, is a professor in the Department of Family Medicine and Community Health at the University of Massachusetts Medical School where she trains family medicine residents and psychologists. She completed her Ph.D. in clinical psychology at Virginia Tech in 1998. She writes and presents extensively about integrated care clinician well-being. Outside of work, she enjoys being a mom of two incredible kids, anything in the woods, meditation, reading, and dark chocolate.

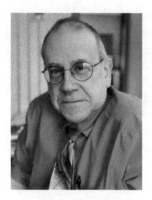

David Conway MD, FACOG, is a semi-retired OB/GYN currently working part-time at a VA Hospital in Manchester, NH, after retiring from the faculty of the NH-Dartmouth Family Medicine Residency in 2016. He graduated from Albany Medical College in 1986 and completed his residency at Hartford Hospital in 1990. He finds immeasurable joy in his children and grandchildren. This is his first publication.

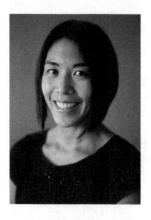

Sarah Gerrish MD, is a health curator. She joined the faculty at the Family Medicine Residency of Idaho as the Kuna clinic Medical Director to further its mission to change health disparities in a meaningful way. At the University of Washington medical school, she emphasized in global/underserved healthcare and now advocates for cultural humility in all settings. Her spouse and sons share her love for climbing and skiing.

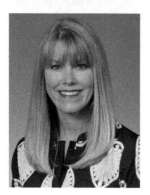

Angela L. Lamson PhD, LMFT, is a Professor in the Medical Family Therapy doctoral program and Marriage and Family Therapy Masters program at East Carolina University. She completed her doctorate in Marriage and Family Therapy at Iowa State University. Outside of work she enjoys raising an amazing son and traveling with her incredible husband.

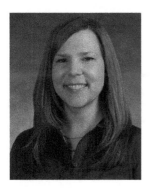

Jackie Williams-Reade PhD, LMFT, is an Associate Professor at Loma Linda University in Loma Linda, CA. She completed a Ph.D. in Medical Family Therapy from East Carolina University in 2011 and a post-doctoral fellowship in pediatric palliative care at Johns Hopkins University in 2012. Outside of work she enjoys long talks with her husband and friends, walking nearby trails with her dog, baking, and watching reality TV.

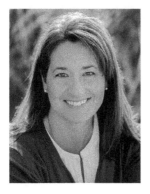

Juli Larsen BS, C-MI, is a meditation instructor in Grand Junction, CO. She completed her undergraduate work at Brigham Young University, majoring in Health Promotions. She enjoys philosophical conversations with her husband, discussing good books with her 5 children, and spending precious quiet time swimming and gardening.

Clinician as Patient

Electronic supplementary material The online version of this chapter (https://doi.org/10.1007/978-3-030-46274-1_5) contains supplementary material, which is available to authorized users.

Advice

Colleen T. Fogarty

A fellow survivor leans in,

and tells me:

    "Count backwards from today to your diagnosis date.

    That's how long it's gonna take—

    at least—

    to begin to feel anything like your old self again…"

I'm definitely a numbers person,

But haven't been able to face

    this counting, calendar exercise

Terrified

the numbers will lie yet again…

The Medicine Box

Aimee Burke Valeras

"What's your Medic Alert bracelet for?" he asked pointedly. He was a tall white man, whose name badge said "Director" and who instantly struck me as the kind of person who didn't think being tall, white, and male had anything to do with his journey to that position. It was my first day in a new job. I looked down at this piece of jewelry that had, without my permission, told this stranger something about me that I had no intention of sharing.

"Your bracelet," he pointed dramatically, as though I didn't know what a bracelet was, "What's it say?" I lingered in silence as he stared at me waiting. I wondered which piece of myself to give him in my answer. A lot was at stake in my response.

My new job was as an "Integrated Behavioral Health Clinician," shortened to "IBHC," which still didn't exactly roll off the tongue. I was bequeathed a small desk in a closet-like room with three other people in the back corner of a dilapidated building full of stale air. The building housed a community health center where a couple dozen family medicine residents learned how to be the kind of physicians that can ideally address mental health and economic deprivation in addition to ear aches and chronic diabetes. In other words, I was a little fish of a social worker in a massive sea of physicians, an invertebrate in an ocean of sharks, charged with teaching the neglected stepsisters of clear-cut medical algorithms, like depression, domestic violence, child abuse, suicidality, and trauma. I had purposefully avoided long flowing skirts and big earrings so as not to look too social-worker-ish, so as not to stand out; but my simple silver bracelet gave me away.

This bracelet had been on my wrist for 19 years, only taken off to add ringlets so it would fit my growing wrist between childhood and adolescence. I was given the bracelet, shiny and delicate, in May of 1986, a few weeks after my father went to a community hospital for a hernia repair—a day surgery that turned into a two-month ICU experience. In the midst of my father's operation, he had a reaction to an ingredient in general anesthesia, succinylcholine, which triggered malignant hyperthermia, a life-threatening condition. The relatively rare MH reaction provided his long string of doctors with the missing piece of a puzzle that tied his many other symptoms together—muscle weakness, winged shoulder blades, droopy eyelids, awkward gait—and led to a diagnosis of muscular dystrophy. My six-year-old mind did not register how close we had come to losing him all together, and I certainly did not understand the impact of the words *Muscular Dystrophy* when those same doctors labeled me with the diagnosis just weeks later. I only knew I had a new bracelet with a charm the shape of an eye. One side was adorned with red letters and a tiny snake wrapped around a scalpel, the other with the careful words: "MALIGNANT HYPERTHERMIA. USE ANESTHETIC PRECAUTIONS."

I had always worn that bracelet like a badge; it had been described to me as the difference between life and death. As I got older, it served as a conversation starter, an icebreaker, an impetus to share my father's story—it was miraculous after all. In the midst of his operation, his body had become rigid as his temperature skyrocketed to 113° Fahrenheit. His heart stopped and the surgical team administered CPR for 16 min.

My father was 32 years old and did not have a Do Not Resuscitate order. They needed my mother, his health care proxy, to give permission for them to stop. They pumped his chest, while one nurse searched for dantrolene, the only treatment available to reverse MH, which coincidentally happened to be in the hospital because of a training on this very issue one day prior, and while another nurse frantically searched for my mother, finding her sprawled comfortably in the lawn in the courtyard of the hospital lazily looking for four-leaf clovers. They described to her his hopeless prognosis—widowhood and single parenthood. She sobbed her assent to stop pumping his chest, just as the cold blanket brought his body temperature down, the breathing tube made it past his crooked nose bones, the dantrolene took effect, and his heart restarted on its own. He survived. This was a good story; I relished the drama, the climax, the awe of my audience.

But here in the medical world, this deceptive bracelet was Morse Code communicating a secret to my new coworkers. Unlike most of my nonmedical audiences, this building full of physicians could quickly deduce that malignant hyperthermia is often linked to neuromuscular disease. I wasn't ashamed of my diagnosis of muscular dystrophy; rather it is very much a part of my identity. I did, however, consciously draw a boundary around my personal medical story so I could focus on establishing myself as a medical professional first. My desire to "pass" as nondisabled was tinged with guilt, recognizing that my visibly disabled peers do not get this privilege, but taking this job as "Dr. Valeras" (albeit in the marginalized behavioral health department), after spending my life on the other side of the table as a patient to a great many specialists, placed me in the unique position to be a covert spy in enemy territory, a sheep in wolves' clothing.

Dr. Tall White Guy was still looking at my Medic Alert bracelet and I answered: "I'm allergic to nosy people." He laughed awkwardly, but he didn't let it go. "What is it for?" he pressed. Searching my name on the Internet would reveal a number of publications in which I openly refer to my diagnosis of muscular dystrophy, based in part, on my doctorate research on the experience of people with disabilities that you can't see by looking at them. It seemed odd to squish myself back "in the closet" as a disabled person, just a month after graduation. But this was my *first* day.

That evening, I pulled out an old medicine box—creaky with spots of rust and covered in stickers. My brother had given it to me one Christmas and it suited me far better than a sparkling ballerina-clad one. I took off my bracelet for the first time in nearly two decades and slipped it into that medicine box indefinitely. That bracelet was symbolically making the line between professional and patient feel blurry.

***

One of the first patients I saw in my IBHC role was "Maria", a 28-year-old woman with cerebral palsy, who walked with a limp and lived in a great deal of pain. Maria's mother was both her main source of support and her worst enemy. Her mother felt heaviness of guilt and sympathy, but she also felt, vociferously, that Maria was malingering and should ignore her pain to maintain her retail job at all costs. Maria had many negative interactions with the medical world, which colored how she viewed all medical professionals—with suspicion, blame, doubt, and mistrust. Maria liked her physician, Dr. Thorton, but to her, his white coat represented every other doctor that had ever let her down. She was referred to me because her anger was getting in the way of her ability to work with her team civilly.

Dr. Thorton paged me to join his office visit and as I walked in the door, she was shouting, "*Why in God's name do you have to say febrile when fever gets the point across just fine?*" She accused him of playing chess with her intellect with medical jargon, creating an upper hand in an already unbalanced power differential. While others bristled at her abrasive anger, I found it understandable. She articulated a concept I had recognized and grappled with, but had been unable to put to words: JSL (Jargon as a Second Language). Maria was persistent in calling it out and I liked her instantly.

> "You two, with your perfect pain-free bodies! You will never understand!" I wanted to tell Maria that I do, in fact, understand what it is like to live in pain.

Maria seemed like the kind of person I would become friends with if I met her in any other context. She was close to my age, enjoyed writing, listened to my favorite bands, and liked the same food. When I would shop in the store where I knew she worked I would feel both hope and dread at the prospect of seeing her, because I didn't know how we would be outside the therapy room. Would we, in an aisle between cleaners and mops, lapse into the kind of chitchat that friends engage in, when the barrier of a coffee table is removed?

Maria was stuck on the idea that no one on her health care team understood what it is like to live in pain. The most repetitive and exasperated sentiment she expressed to Dr. Thorton and me was, "You two, with your perfect pain-free bodies! You will never understand!" I wanted to tell Maria that I do, in fact, understand what it is like to live in pain. I was going to share with her a snippet of my story—my diagnosis of MD, a childhood of surgeries, the pain I live with today. I wanted her to know just enough information to get unstuck her from her notion that I didn't understand, so that we could engage in a therapeutic relationship that moved forward.

In comparison to my doctor and nurse colleagues, my boundaries seem fairly rigid when it comes to self-disclosure. But even within the Behavioral Health Department, there are subspecialties—clinical psychologist, mental health counselor, social worker, marriage and family therapist—and each draws a unique line in the sand about how much personal self can be brought into the therapy room. But all clinicians should explore the purpose for disclosing personal information to clients—is it for increasing intimacy or is it self-serving? In other words, could I be absolutely sure that I wanted to tell her a chapter of my illness narrative to move Maria forward and allow her to see I'm on her side, but *not* to center my story in our relationship? I discussed this inner monologue with Dr. Thorton, wondering about his opinion. He surprised me by sharing his own childhood diagnosis of juvenile rheumatoid arthritis. He too experienced many medical encounters and pain at a young age. Together we decided to share these pieces of ourselves with Maria, and it *did* turn out to be a catalyst to her seeing us as her team and on her side, rather than her enemy.

Dr. Thorton and I both had more in common with Maria than she realized, but we also discovered a shared disability identity with each other. Knowing about each other's "hidden disabilities"—aspects of our identities, which are equally as formative and important as our genders, ethnicities, religions, political perspectives—made our working relationship more authentic. My own wrist, where my Medic Alert bracelet used to dangle, is a reminder of the two selves that a health care provider creates when he or she is also a patient. Why is disability within our own ranks so taboo?

We shared the story of our work with Maria with a group of colleagues to prompt a discussion about our differing boundaries and how it shapes the decisions we make with patients and our relationships with them. When I shared how I disclosed my diagnosis of MD to Maria to further our clinical relationship, I was actually disclosing my disability to my colleagues, by means of this story itself. The way the room of medical colleagues looked at me after this disclosure was intangible, but I interpreted pity dancing on their expressions; maybe even disgust, but not because they look down upon self-disclosure. I've listened as physicians have shared graphic particulars of their own vasectomies; delicious details of their children's excreting warts; or triumphs and tribulations with crash diets. I think the indignation was the revelation that I had a *real* enemy of a diagnosis—not one that gets cured in the neat equation that Western medicine is designed for: *yesterday I was healthy, today I am sick, tomorrow* (with heroic efforts and prescriptions) *I will be healthy again* (Frank 1995). Unyielding, uncurable, unpreventable, unstoppable disability makes physicians really uncomfortable, particularly when it shows up on the wrong side of the desk. The dichotomy between the able-bodied and the disabled, however false, is encouraged and embraced. Able-bodied, not disabled. Doctor, not patient. As long as disability is different, exceptional, uncommon, an outlier, health care providers can rest in the comfort that one's current physical or mental state is permanent. In revealing my own disability to my colleagues, I was representing the fragility of their able-bodiedness; the fallacy of their role as provider, never patient.

Arthur Frank, in *The Wounded Storyteller*[1], announced a "call to arms," luring health care providers who have a personal experience with bodily infallibility and mortality to allow their solidly constructed boundary to drop, if only temporarily, to offer this part of themselves to certain patients. Their "club membership" allows them specific knowledge of "club secrets" and to collude together about this shared understanding may allow patients to feel that they are not alone.

***

It was a beautiful autumn day. Sun was streaming through the multicolored trees, as they freed their leaves one at a time in coordination with the soft breeze. It was a day of excruciating pain radiating up and down my taut leg muscles. When the pain is like this, it is indescribable and so very incongruous with the beauty around me. I was running late for work, and I knew there was a young man waiting for me there, newly diagnosed with multiple sclerosis and struggling to wrap his mind around what this means for who he is as an athlete, as a father, as a person. It was important to me and for him that I barrel through my pain and make it to this appointment, to sit with his anguish. But on my way out the door, I paused and retreated. I creaked open my eccentric and charming medicine box and gingerly took my Medic Alert bracelet out. It was cold in my fingers, but so familiar; it had been waiting for me. I slipped it back on, and it felt like I was reunited with an old friend.

Go ahead, I whispered into the empty air, *ask me what my Medic Alert bracelet is for. I dare you.*

---

[1]Frank, A. (1995). *The wounded storyteller: Body, illness, and ethics.* Chicago, IL: The University of Chicago Press.

Stuck

Kathryn Hart

You are careful

You are organized, well-trained
follow all the rules, best-practices
You're involved in a *Culture of Safety*
But inevitably...

You will be poked.

In dentistry, everything is sharp -
   teeth, needles, burs
   the bone after an extraction - feel to know if you must smooth
You will be poked.

What to do?

Suddenly an unwilling blood-brother
with a schedule to keep, denial to quell

Some will choose the difficult conversation
   "I have been exposed to your blood."
   "Are you willing to submit to a blood-draw?"

my children...?
my husband...?
my life...?

You were my patient.
Now our relationship is changed
If you give blood to relieve my fears,
it is you who will be taking care of me.

Others will not mention it
...and worry
and stew
for days
for months
For six months, actually, you will not know for sure.
You await your final blood results

Whatever you do, whatever the results,
You are stuck
You will be back touching sharp objects again tomorrow
And careful as you are,
You will be poked.

Embracing Our Origin Stories

R. L. Hughes

"She's a minimizer," my neurologist said bluntly to my tearful mother as I sat with pinhole vision to her right.

"She's always been that way," my mother responded.

I sat silently wondering what was happening to my future before my near-blind eyes. This was a beginning point in my origin story.

***

We're used to hearing the origin stories of superheroes, of the strife and tragedy these characters faced in order to reveal their superpowers. We know Spiderman was inspired by the murder of his uncle, Batman by the murder of his parents, and Superman by the murder of his home planet. But what about the lesser known origin of you and me? The experiences, the reason we came to be as we are today doing exactly what we are doing in this moment. We don't hear about the triumphs of the woman who makes it out of bed after grappling with depression for months. They don't tell you about the man who gets his A1c under control one year after it being a 12.6. These are the moments that harden us to the pains we face in life and make us better able to deal with future challenges and help others do the same. I prefer the origin story of the everyday hero. My origin story led me to my role as medical family therapist—an advocate for patient-centered and whole-person care.

***

I was 20 years old, studying Zoology, with my entire life ahead of me. If only I hadn't been dealing with these "aural migraines," the neurologist called them. I figured something had to go wrong since everything else was working so well.

After a brief spring vacation with my friend, we were headed back to campus, recounting the woes of a hectic semester, and I noticed my vision crackling around the edges. These migraines weren't particularly painful, more of a minor visual annoyance as they shattered my view like broken glass.

As the miles back to campus crept by, my vision grew dimmer and dimmer. Eventually, I was left with no more than an eraser-sized field of vision in both eyes. My friend helped me back to our apartment, and I lay in my bed, waiting and wondering if my vision was going to naturally return.

> These are the moments that harden us to the pains we face in life and make us better able to deal with future challenges and help others do the same.

***

My vision didn't improve, instead crippling vertigo doubled my difficulties, making a simple trip to the bathroom a chaotic and nauseating experience and walking to classes nearly impossible. I thought that if I could just get to class I could pretend things were "normal," even if that meant taking 30 minutes to stagger the 10 minute route. People glared at me like I was intoxicated. After a few weeks of no improvement and the forceful suggestion of my worried parents, I called my neurologist again. He saw me immediately.

My origin story begins when I became a real *patient* for the first time in my life. I went through a whirlwind of invasive tests; I was poked, prodded, and pic-lined with little to no explanation of what was going on; my parents dashing behind me to keep up. The neurologist had his suspicions of my diagnosis but gave us no information, probably fearful of jumping to the wrong conclusion. As a patient I craved for the information that was being withheld. Over the course of two months my neurologist slowly excluded all other explanations for my loss of balance and sight, and finally he concluded that I had multiple sclerosis.

I ricocheted through the next few months after the diagnosis. I dropped out of my school program, but luckily had enough credit hours to graduate. I was asked to resign from my position as residence manager. I uprooted my life to move back home to live with my dad. I was particularly bitter about moving back home because it felt like I had failed my mission of becoming an adult. I had worked so hard to purposefully shape the life I wanted, but here I was, back at home.

***

My rock bottom happened a few months after hitting home. My daily routine was lying in my bed in a dark room watching movies all day. I could absorb myself in the plots, avoid the fact that I felt like my life was directionless, that I was an orphan of fate, a benefactor of misfortune. Then my dad and his wife would come home and ask how my day was. "Fine."

I don't remember the exact turning point, but, as my vision returned a little more each day, I became increasingly restless. I craved direction and purpose in my life. I needed to take a step toward what mattered most to me. I needed to stand up for myself because I was tired of waiting for someone to show up and fix the pieces of my life. After 45 days of spending more than 20 hours a day in my bedroom, I emerged and started to engage with what was outside the walls of my father's house.

I was terrified of resuming my life, fearful that at any moment I would break again, go blind, but I knew that something had to change if I were ever to reclaim any purpose in my life. After evaluating what was really important to me, I discovered that I needed to help other people in some way. My fears were still present, but the urgency to do something important was greater. I needed to be there for someone else. So, I emailed the program director of a Marriage and Family Therapy graduate program. "Do you think someone with a zoology degree can do something like this?" My heart pounded until I received a response shortly after, fearful of the rejection that might tear me apart.

"Well, humans are just animals; aren't they?" he responded.

Over the next two years, I learned and studied the techniques that would help me help others and also reclaim myself. I learned the words "self-efficacy" and "empowerment"—words that I interlace in all of the clinic conversations I have now. I practiced daily mindfulness exercises that allowed me to make space for my traumatic experience. Through this process, I began to make peace with the uprooting of my planned life with each intentional breath. I started eating healthy foods and running daily as a means to target my baseline anxiety. I developed a program that allowed me to cope with what had happened to me and experience my life more fully. I now share these tools with patients on a daily basis because I can offer them from a place of knowing and not just telling.

Near the end of my master's training, I became intrigued by medical family therapy. To me it seemed like medical family therapy encapsulated my experience of being a patient and was a vessel to channel my therapeutic tools in a mean-ingful way. I could be the person that I had needed when I was tumbling recklessly through the testing and medical system and help other patients get through with a glimmer of hope that I lacked in my experience. I wanted to empower others to be their own hero.

And as I finish my doctorate in medical family therapy, I truly believe this is the path that I have carved out for myself. I work at a family medicine residency with physicians, case managers, and nurses to support our patients in indentifying their own strengths and powers as a means for coping with and creating meaning out of illness.

In this process I have found that my own superpower is staying attuned to patients who have heard the word "chronic" or "terminal." I sit with them in the disaster and witness the vulnerability and power of the moment. I listen, I wait, and I am with them, as someone who knows what it feels like to have the future become less certain in an instant. I suspect that my story of finding purpose through illness is not a unique one, but I share it to pay credence to the origin story of the Everyday Hero who often gets overlooked. For some, their trials are overcoming medical and psychiatric symptoms. Others face the challenge of overcoming the medical system itself. But it's the small things we do every day to help ourselves and to help others, that make a better life.

Now tell me, what's your origin story?

There Is More to Life than Work

Tai J. Mendenhall

On paper, I have almost-always looked good. I earned great grades in college, and did anything and everything "extra" that I could—like volunteering on faculty research projects and serving in human-service organizations. In graduate school, I performed in many of the same ways. My doctoral internship in a Psychiatry residency was a natural culmination of this momentum. Eighty-hour work weeks represented a "standard" that I had become familiar with as par-for-the-course in Academia (generally) and Medicine (specifically).

When I began my first assistant professor post, I was well-equipped for the roles and lifestyle that a large Research-1 university sought in its "best and brightest." Professional value was (is) measured by hours spent at work, gallons of coffee consumed, numbers of papers published, dollars secured for scholarship, and generating "value" by seeing as many patients as humanly possible. I hit the ground running…

Rationalizing the Problem

I was not ignorant to the unhealthy nature of my lifestyle; I just did not see any other way to function. The superstars who preceded me were doing the same things—working long hours, living on fast- and/or prepackaged-foods, and going strong in a tireless state of caffeinated-focus. I did not know much about their personal lives, but understood that many of them had been married and divorced. They preached the merits of good diets, sleep hygiene, and date-nights to patients —but never followed their own counsel.

And me? I knew that I was on the right path. It sucked that I, too, had to experience the pain of divorce in order to follow it, though. The fact that I had gone from a once svelte physique to being 50 + pounds overweight wasn't good, either. I recall being initially resistant to going on blood pressure meds during my 30s, but rationalized it on the grounds that things would improve once I was promoted with tenure. Then I could walk-the-walk with good self-care.

I told myself—and others—these things, but I never really believed it. My life's work would forever be in service to others. Their health, their relationships, and their happiness. At what cost? My own, of course. Somehow, over time, I had internalized this as okay.

A Wake-Up Call

I will never forget how the wisdom of work/life balance came to me in a manner that "stuck." I was sitting in a large conference room for a grand-rounds presentation. The presenter came with visual aids. His talk was going to center on what many already understand as a relatively well-known, albeit rarely practiced, metaphor. The following is how I experienced—and internalized—its wisdom.

As I got settled-in for the presentation (junk food and coffee in-hand), the presenter set a large mason jar down on a table at the front of the room. Then he laid out some large rocks. Then he poured gravel onto the table, and finally, sand. *Okay, that's a bit messy*, I thought.

"All of these ingredients will fit into this jar," the speaker said. "But only if you put them in in the right order."

My colleagues and I looked around the room at each other for a moment. *This isn't really a very hard question*, I thought. *Big stuff first, right?*

Somebody finally said what everyone was thinking: "You put the rocks in first. Then the gravel, and then the sand."

The speaker agreed. "That's right! First the rocks," and he put them into the mason jar. "Then the gravel goes in around the rocks." He put the gravel in. "And then the sand." We all watched for a couple of minutes as he scooped up the sand and poured it into the jar—shaking it a bit to make each scoop settle into the remaining spaces.

None of this seemed very life-changing to me at first. *Of course you put the ingredients in in that order*, I thought. *Just like Study Skills 101: first do your big assignments, and then do the little ones.*

"Okay, now think about this jar as a metaphor for your day. Or your life." He paused for a moment to let that sink in. "What are the biggest things for you? The most important things? The rocks?"

Several hands went up.

"My case notes," somebody said. Everyone laughed. I could certainly relate to that one.

Others offered other—better—ideas. Some talked about their spouses and/or kids. Some talked about their faith and/or church.

"What about yourselves?" the speaker asked. "Can you include the person who you are with for 24 hours each day on your list of rocks?" It is still amazing to me that nobody had thought of this until then. Things like exercising, or reading a novel for fun.

Where in the world does anybody find time for that?, I thought.

The speaker went on. "Gravel? This is stuff that is important, but the world won't end if you don't get to it today."

Somebody asked, "Like getting the oil changed in your car?"

"That's a great example! You need to do it when your '10% oil life' light comes on, but you'll probably be okay doing it later in the week if you cannot fit it in today."

"And sand? What, diagnostically, will nobody really give a damn about? Or even remember a day or two from now?"

Lots of examples here. People called out things like folding their laundry, washing dishes, and reading emails.

"But how many of you do it all backwards?", our speaker asked. "How many of you run around like the mad, crazy-busy, over-scheduled people—checking off your to-do lists all day long—only to come home every night exhausted? Sorry honey, not tonight. Missing your kid's ballgame (again)? One more time, not going to the gym?"

At this point, I began to feel uncomfortable. And besides, I needed to get back to clinic.

"How many of you are doing great work, professionally, but are watching your own physical bodies get out-of-shape?"

I looked down at my obese belly. I had my arms crossed, resting on it like some sort of biological table attached at my midriff. I couldn't even remember the last time I went running. *I used to love running.*

"How many of your relationships are dying of neglect?"

I guess it doesn't matter that I'm fat, I thought. *It's not like I'm on-the-prowl, anyway.* The last couple of people I tried to have long-term relationships with had left me. *And what difference does it make if I work so much?*, I thought. *I go home to an empty house.*

"Well, at least you're caught up with emails and Facebook," the speaker said.

As many laughed (with varying degrees of discomfort), I recall sitting there, stunned. A bit ashamed, even. I was doing everything backwards. No wonder the only thing I was good at was my work. And no wonder—despite having achieved so many professional accolades—I was so dangerously out-of-shape, so intolerably lonely, and so very unhappy.

It was on that day that I realized that there is more to life than work.

Responding to the Problem

The very next morning—and on every morning since—I woke up and asked myself, *What are my rocks*? The person who I am with 24 hours each day is a rock. And that means that I take time to take care of him—whether it's going running or to the gym, taking the long way home on my motorcycle, or reading a novel before bedtime. My career—of course, is a rock. And when I am there, I work hard. But I leave it there when I go home. I deleted the software from my laptop that allowed me access to my case files off-site. I re-arranged my home "office" to be a library, instead, and I only do relaxing and non-work things there. As I lost weight and gained better mental health, I found love again. We married—and our union is a rock. I honor her—us—with my time, energy, and whole self. Every day.

When I can squeeze it in, I take care of gravel. My car's oil is fine. And sand? Whenever I get behind with emails, laundry, or yard work—it's amazing how somehow, some way, I always get caught up.

All of these things are processes, not events. They require vigilant attention. And there have, indeed, been times when I have found myself working too much again. I notice this when I "haven't had time" to go to the gym lately, or when my pants are getting tight. I notice it, too, when something professionally good happens, like winning a grant or having a paper accepted for publication, and I don't feel happy or excited about it. When these things happen, I re-ground, I re-prioritize. I work to reclaim my health, and all of the biopsychosocial/spiritual things that this means. *What are my rocks*?

My productivity at work, almost paradoxically, has improved. I achieved tenure several years ago. I consistently secure funding to advance my scholarship. I regularly disseminate new knowledge through my writing and teaching. I do effective clinical work. But I don't have a biological table to rest my arms on anymore. I don't go home to an empty house.

And I am happy.

From Zero to Four Under Two

Grace Pratt and Jonathan B. Wilson

Grace: We may have married at twenty, but we persevered through eight years, three moves, and six academic degrees (between us) before we started trying for a baby. Two nearly finished doctorate Medical Family Therapists set out to achieve a pregnancy with all the gusto you'd expect from a couple of researchers, but I quickly knew something was wrong. I tracked my cycle and basal body temperature and analyzed for months, with no sign of ovulation. My program of research centered on childbearing decision making, infertility, and reproductive trauma —an expertise that weighed heavily on me as we started fertility testing, then treatment. All my knowledge and research gave us no control over biology.

Finally, we sat in the office of the Reproductive Endocrinologist, a surreal juxtaposition of data and lived experience converging within that moment. The plan was simple, stepwise, and brought back some semblance of control. We trudged through a couple of failed procedures, but then to our surprise, I only needed medically induced ovulation to become pregnant. A healthy, straightforward pregnancy brought us Henry, who simultaneously exhausted and delighted us. When he turned one, we decided to try again. This time, our first medicated cycle resulted in pregnancy, and early genetic testing found male DNA. We prepared our home and our hearts for another son.

Jonathan: One bright Wednesday morning, we went to our doctor's office for our first ultrasound. Henry turned fifteen months old that day, and there was a snap of cool mid-October air as we'd left the house. Grace lay on the ultrasound table and I stood by her side, our eyes trained on the monitor, expecting to confirm what we already knew (another boy), hoping he was healthy. Nearly immediately, our ultrasound technician's words rang out: "Are you guys ready for this? You're having twins! No, wait, it's triplets!" Our mouths dropped, tears flowed, and I had to sit down. When we saw they were all boys, Grace, through tears, laughed "Our house is going to smell so bad!" We weren't prepared for this. Our care team wasn't prepared for this. Monochorionic triplets are so rare that none of our providers had ever seen them. Our ultrasound technician asked if she could take a photo of our ultrasound to share with her colleagues.

Our lives, in that moment, changed catastrophically. We needed space to process. Instead of going back to the waiting room, we waited for our appointment in an empty exam room so that we could decompress in privacy. We cried. We hugged. We called family. The initial shock was overwhelming. Unfortunately, our OBGYN was out of the office that day, but his nurse practitioner was so kind and beautifully conveyed empathy toward us. She'd just found out she was expecting twins herself. We knew we had a long road ahead—multiple visits with maternal fetal medicine, more ultrasounds than we could count—watching our babies closely. Waiting to see if they'd be okay. All three shared a single placenta, which multiplied the possible complications.

Grace: Everyone we knew was shocked. We walked out of the clinic and sat in the car making phone calls for about an hour—including one to our realtor, because our house was now too small. Henry was really too young to understand we'd be bringing one baby home, much less three. Many people who we told even thought we were joking. The residency clinic where I teach is less than a half a mile from my obstetrician's office, and by the time I wandered back over there in a daze, they were just starting our daily didactic session over lunch. I walked up to a physician attending colleague, handed him the ultrasound and asked—"How many babies do you see here?" Waves of shock and excitement rippled through my colleagues and the residents, but I could also see concern and fear for us on their faces.

We expected that everything in our lives had to be rearranged, but we didn't actually know what life would be like after the babies were born. One big issue was a lack of local family support. We lived in Oklahoma, away from all of our family support in Texas, because of our careers. Dual academic career families typically have to live where the opportunity is, and we'd been so fortunate to find an MFT faculty position and a MedFT residency teaching position within an hour of one another. We both loved our jobs and had worked hard to build our careers to this point, but we also felt we were on tenuous ground—how would my 50 min commute affect our family? What kind of childcare situation could we find that would accommodate Jonathan's evening classes? How could we maintain the trajectories of our nascent careers with this fundamental change in the demands of our family? And, beyond just the demands of having three babies, their risk of complications was high. What kind of special medical needs would they have? Perhaps most frustratingly, we couldn't answer any of those questions; no one could. They hung in the air, ever-present but unresolved.

Jonathan: We knew about the triplets for only 14 weeks before they were born. Our doctors predicted we wouldn't have to decide when to deliver— that triplets always show us when it is time. Grace was hospitalized on bed rest for two weeks with pre-term labor, and we grew accustomed to our daily routine of ultrasounds, biophysical profiles of each baby, hospital food, and less than comfortable sleeping arrangements. One morning, our smallest baby's heartrate was unpredictable. Our OBGYN came to the room and watched the ultrasound; he didn't like what he saw, and the consultant agreed. Reverse cord flow meant Alex was telling us it was time.

We were launched into an organized frenzy of activity. Nurses and doctors flooded in and out of our room. The anesthesiologist introduced himself to us, quickly explained what was going to happen while the nurses prepped Grace for surgery, and then we rolled to the operating room. I was directed to a holding area to scrub in and wait until Grace's spinal block was administered to numb her for the cesarean section. As I entered the operating room, I took in the crowd of people—there were at least five doctors (one anesthesiologist, two OBYGNs, two neonatologists), and probably a dozen others—nurses, respiratory therapists, students. Everyone was waiting with electric anticipation. Teams were assigned to Grace and each individual baby. I sat by Grace's head as her OBGYN began the C-section 1:12 pm, 1:13 pm, 1:13 pm—within two minutes, our babies arrived. I caught glimpses of each baby for a brief moment as they were handed off to their own medical teams. Grace wanted me to tell her everything: Do they look alike? Do they have hair? Are they breathing? I did my best to answer as the action continued around me. None of the boys cried, but the doctors told us they looked good and they were strong. They were whisked across the hall to the NICU, each with his own team working to stabilize him.

As soon as I could, I made my way to the NICU while Grace's surgery was completed. I wasn't able to hold any of the babies yet (I wouldn't have done so without Grace even if I could), but I met my three boys for the first time—each so tiny, yet so perfect. The boys were each in a neonatal incubator. They were intubated, and their IVs were in their heads because the veins in their arms were too small. Their skin was very thin from being born so early—they looked red and you could see their veins running along their bodies. As I looked past the medical interventions, the detail that stood out to me was that each one had fine blonde hair all over their heads just like their big brother Henry. I was amazed at how prepared our medical team was—for a birth that none of them would likely ever see again in their careers. Each person had a job, a purpose. Even though I knew we had a long road ahead, I felt safe and confident that our boys would be okay.

Grace: We settled into a routine of NICU visits, gifted meals, pumping, and commuting. Our days were spent weighing diapers and learning to feed preemies and holding skin to skin, while our evenings were time with Henry and managing home. Jonathan returned to classes when the spring semester started. We began again finding a balance of work and home, and now hospital. Every morning I joined the team rounding on the babies, and every evening before I fell asleep I called the night nurse for an update. Three tiny boys grew, and we celebrated each milliliter drank and every ounce gained. For babies born at 29 weeks they were doing remarkably well, but each boy had setbacks—an early infection for Alex, a hole that wasn't closing in James's heart, and fluctuating bilirubin for Luke. Our professional lives moved forward while standing still. Jonathan's colleagues took over all his responsibilities except teaching—he had no committee service, no advisees, and no supervisees. While I had continued to work and did supervision from my hospital bed on bedrest, my 8-week maternity leave started when the babies were born.

The scariest day came when they were one month and one day old. When I arrived to visit, a nurse I hadn't met before told me James was showing signs of infection. They'd stopped his feeds, started antibiotics, and were watching his abdomen closely. The curtain was drawn around his isolette, and they'd moved him away from his brothers. Posted signs demanded isolation procedures and contact precautions. I donned a gown and a mask and gloves and stood by his bed, reaching through a hole to touch him because he was too weak for me to hold. "I'm so emotionally depleted," I wrote to friends. "I'm on empty."

When his doctor came, I was too terrified to ask the question I most wanted to know. The irony isn't lost on me that as a MedFT teaching in a family medicine residency program, a significant part of my role is helping doctors and patients communicate. I empower patients to have the agency to raise concerns with their medical team, and I give new physicians language to use to discuss life and death scenarios with patients and their families. Yet, in this moment, the grip of fear for my own child was too strong for me to speak.

Although I still didn't speak the words, my tears and silences and hesitations must have been loud enough. "Tell me what you're afraid of. If you say it out loud, we can walk through it together." Her compassion bolstered me to find the words, "Necrotizing enterocolitis." NEC is a complication that most often occurs in premature babies where part of the intestine becomes inflamed and can die. The condition is associated with severe morbidity and mortality, and I personally knew a mother whose son had died from developing NEC. "Yes," she said. "I'm watching for that. We're monitoring everything, doing all the necessary intervention. If it is NEC, we're already doing everything we can." Once more, we were left to wait. After a few days, his infection resolved without consequence. My fear—although unspeakably terrifying—came to nothing.

Jonathan: Finally, after seven weeks, it was time to come home. Everything was prepared—Grace's mom in town, the cribs assembled, the car seats ready to go. The night before the babies' hospital discharge, Green Day came to town, and we decided to capitalize on our last date opportunity for a while. I had always loved the band, and it felt right as a last celebration. The next week would be spring break for my classes, and Grace had one week of maternity leave left, so we had a week together as a family before we had to start trying to balance three babies and a toddler at home, two careers, and extreme sleep deprivation and fatigue. We stood in the arena and familiar lyrics washed over us as we held hands, looked at each other, and tried to soak in the moment.

> Another turning point, a fork stuck in the road.
> Time grabs you by the wrist, directs you where to go
> So make the best of this test, and don't ask why
> It's not a question, but a lesson learned in time.
>
> Take the photographs and still-frames in your mind
> Hang them on a shelf in good health and good time...
>
> For what it's worth, it was worth all the while.
> It's something unpredictable, but in the end it's right.
> I hope you had the time of your life.
>
> Green Day

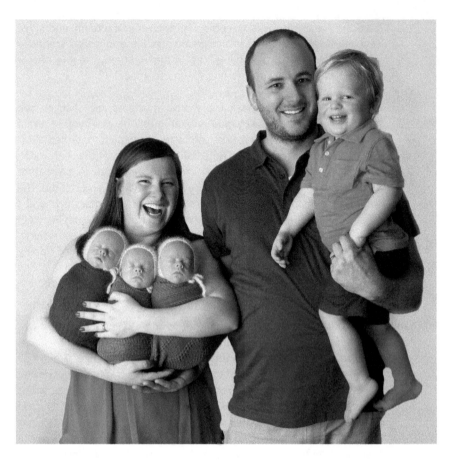

Caught in a Culture of Shame

Samantha Pelican Monson

I am a mother and wife, sister, daughter, auntie, and dear friend. I am also a psychologist who has worked in primary care for over a decade. Finally, I am a 39-year-old woman with cystic fibrosis. The intersection of these myriad identities includes the fact that I'm "sick" and also "healthy" at the same time. This paradox has created confusion for me throughout my life, including in the context of my profession.

Cystic fibrosis (CF) is a rare genetic disease that primarily impacts the respiratory and digestive systems. Its genetics are very complicated, so no two CF patients have exactly the same symptom profile or prognosis. I was diagnosed with CF at a year old. Lucky for me, my parents ensured I had excellent medical care and did all the recommended treatments. This, combined with several scientific break-throughs, means that I have been able to live a "normal" life.

Because CF is a chronic disease for which there is no cure, its impact on my career is ongoing and ever-changing. There are day-to-day challenges. I do an hour of medical treatments every morning and another hour every night, which sand-wiched around a busy day at the safety net clinic where I work gets exhausting. There are logistical challenges. For example, CF requires high caloric intake both for nutrition and glucose control, which is always in the back of my mind as consults crowd my lunch hour and leave no room for even quick snack breaks. There are system challenges. For example, although I function as a consultant for any patient who walks through the door, I have to be very careful about exposure to even mild infections. And those are just the start of the challenges. I could go on and on with stories about patients' reactions to the shrink knowing *a lot* about their respiratory meds, the time I overheard a precepting conversation about why someone with compromised health would want to have children (I was trying to get pregnant at the time), and more.

So with all these challenges unique to my practice setting, why have I stayed? Because I had the privilege of experiencing the power of high-quality team-based care as a patient long, long before I knew what it was.

I was 11 years old, sitting cross-legged in my hospital bed and chatting-it-up with my favorite nurse named Olivia. The sun filtered in through the greeting card collage I'd taped to the window as well wishes had arrived over the previous weeks. I was making plans to go down the hall to the patient activity room for a craft before the respiratory therapist arrived for my next airway clearance procedure. This was a typical scene from what CF patients call "tune ups," when we require more intensive intervention for lung infections. Except this one was about to go wrong...a 105° fever, profound fatigue and delirium, and a diagnosis by bone marrow testing of neutropenia. Under more physical and emotional stress than any child can reasonably endure, I started hallucinating in the middle of the night and the psychiatrist was called. He slowly pulled me back into a more peaceful reality as my medical situation improved. He worked with my pulmonology team to conceptualize my experience as a trauma, and to point to earlier medical traumas that should also be incorporated into my ongoing care plan. From then on, each of my CF appointments included a social worker who helped me make sense of my illness experiences, so I could be better prepared to face the next challenge.

I was drawn to health psychology because of my experiences as a patient, and yet those same experiences add challenges to how I conceptualize myself everyday. My identity as a patient is undeniably strong, no matter how much I may abhor that reality. And yet I have stepped into the role of treating patients, essentially putting me on the other side of the clinical interview. One way I have grown to manage this is to carefully guard CF as a secret. I told almost no one with whom I went to graduate school and then no one with whom I started working. I worried I would be viewed as a patient—a "them"—and would not be accepted as an "us" by the teams on which I worked. I feared being thought of as weak. I was concerned about somehow being a burden to those who already carried the burdens of so many patients.

Here and there, I have started to disclose CF to colleagues. Like any secret, the weight of maintaining it can increase with time, and sometimes transparency is the most responsible course of action. Although I've never had a negative experience disclosing CF to a coworker, I remain reluctant to do so. A big reason for this is that there is no culture of pride or acceptance in being a patient among healthcare providers. Much of this messaging is implicit, essentially micro-aggressions toward the *dis*abled population. For example, one of the medical providers was in a serious car accident on the way to work one morning. Injured, she still arrived to start seeing patients. Although the medical director sent her home, she returned after lunch, bandaged and with an ice pack on her arm. I watched as everyone "high fived" her for limiting her patient status to a mere four hours. What if instead she had been empowered to take care of herself, as we encourage our patients to do?

It saddens me that this culture of shame around patient status persists. I see opportunity, as we all rely on relationships to sustain and enable us to make a difference, and those same relationships could support a colleague with CF or any other "wound." And my experiences with disclosure have not in themselves been negative. On the contrary, in response to learning about CF, I am often noted to have a unique capacity for empathy, an extra strong work ethic, and persistence in bringing about change. So perhaps part of my "job" is to use these to help create a healthier culture, to break the conspiracy of silence that further stigmatizes helping professionals who themselves require help.

A Terrifying and Altering Reversal

Jamie E. Banker

Shock, fear, tears, everything seemed surreal
Time stood still, diagnosis revealed
Trained as a therapist to assess and treat
Now I am put in the patient seat

I listened to the doctor—words I could not believe
I questioned his accuracy, I started to grieve
I was worried and hurried, needed time to process
How could I decide, my thinking obsessed

Injunctions, infusions watched my body distort
Estranged from my life I grew weary and short
I cannot accept it, I was naked and helpless
The growing discomfort I felt was relentless

But I still showed up despite how discouraged
The faces in front of me helped me find courage
These faces were always my constant, my routine
They were my certain when certainty was unseen

I see my work freshly thanks to all they have done
They showed me the provider I want to become
So I copy their efforts with all my ability
How they listened and taught with gentle humility

A rare intimacy I will not forget feeling
From them I learned how to inspire healing.

An MFT's Journey Through Infertility, Motherhood, and Postpartum Depression and Anxiety

Tania Riosvelasco

May 12, 2015.

"He was born on May 1st, 2015 at 2:25 a.m. Twenty-four hours of labor from when my water broke to when he gave his first cry—loud and clear, with such force that it took my breath away.

He's been in this world for eleven days now and it has been surreal. Beautiful. Tiresome. But a blessing in all the senses of the word.

Every tear, every heartache, every empty promise that came month after month... I can say now that it was worth it. Worth the waiting and the uncertainty; the sadness and the loneliness of the journey. This journey that I undertook in the quest to find him. A journey that has been one of the most painful experiences of my life.

But he finally came. I am so grateful that I didn't give up."

2019

I wrote this six years ago when my eldest son was born; in the midst of a postpartum bliss of finally becoming a mother, of birthing a child. My child. My son. A wish to grow my family that went unfulfilled for almost three years before, and finally achieving a successful pregnancy through the process of *in vitro fertilization* (IVF). I did not know at that time that the challenges of infertility were still not over. I was not aware that the underlying anxiety that I had been experiencing since starting this infertility journey would eventually turn into postpartum anxiety and depression. And I didn't know how it would also have a ripple effect in my marriage.

I started my infertility journey with such hope and naiveté, and the end result of bringing my son home was worth every second of it. But I wish I had not been so alone in this journey; I wish I had had a therapist, or even my doctor, supporting and acknowledging the hardship of this experience.

2010

I was 24 years old and was a recently graduated Marriage and Family Therapist intern working at a family medicine clinic in San Diego, CA. My husband and I had decided that we wanted to start a family, and we were aware that this might require medical intervention as he had been diagnosed a few years back with male factor infertility. It didn't seem too daunting of a process at the time. We found a fertility clinic and requested an appointment. I clearly remember being in the doctor's office and being told something along the lines of, "You're young and healthy. It should be fairly easy for you to get pregnant. There's no need to worry." Those words would become my mantra in the months and years ahead, both in the USA and Germany where my treatments took place to help me cope with the pervasive sadness that I felt before finally achieving a successful pregnancy.

2010–2012

These years were spent in a state that could be best described as limbo. A fine balance between not being pregnant but managing my life around the possibility of becoming pregnant. My treatment started with a couple of intrauterine inseminations (IUIs) attempts and ended with a frozen embryo transfer (FET), and it lasted about four years. The moments in between significantly affected my emotional and mental health, as I found myself feeling a pervasive sadness and sense of hopelessness that did not lift until I heard and saw the first heartbeat. It then got replaced with an anxious feeling that did not leave until I felt my first born's first kicks. And even then, I did not feel able to fully relax.

Looking back, I wonder why the mental and emotional aspect of my treatment was not taken more into consideration. "It's normal," was often what I heard in reply to my concerns. I had a lingering, uncomfortable feeling that the whole process resembled more a factory line up: couples unable to get pregnant naturally, going into the fertility clinic, given a treatment plan, and a pregnancy would happen. Easy, and almost effortless.

My journey included two failed IUIs, an extreme allergic reaction to progesterone that made it almost impossible to continue with the first treatment, one failed IVF cycle that required an emergency hospitalization as I developed ovarian hyperstimulation syndrome (OHSS), a surprise natural pregnancy that turned out to be ectopic and required emergency life-saving surgery. And finally, a frozen embryo transfer (FET) that did end up being a successful pregnancy of a single baby boy.

2013–2016

Both pregnancies (the first one that took so much work to achieve, and my second one that happened naturally and miraculously) were riddled with worry and fear from day one. I remember crying every single day during the first trimester, feeling anxious that I might lose the pregnancy. I remember feeling this incredibly debilitating worry that would consume my thoughts and energy. In both pregnancies, this extreme anxiety lessened after I started feeling the baby's movement but it didn't completely go away.

The postpartum period after my second pregnancy, however, was much different from my first one. There was this constant underlying anxiety present, in the form of intrusive thoughts and physical symptoms. I would worry when taking the train that my stroller might accidentally slip forward and fall into the train tracks. Or I would be hypervigilant while in the kitchen because of the fear that a knife might slip and hurt one of my children. It did not matter that the knives were tucked safely away. I also started to avoid looking at myself in the mirror. Looking at my reflection made me feel so overwhelmed and unhappy.

The lack of sleep made this experience increasingly worse. I thought I was being successful in managing this anxiety—I practiced deep breathing, identified and challenged my negative thoughts and cognitive distortions, I reached out to my group of friends for support, I talked to my husband, and I tried to sleep and maintain a healthy lifestyle. My youngest was born in late February, and it was about late December, during the holidays back in my home country Mexico, where one day I felt like I couldn't breathe. I literally could not catch a breath and I felt incredibly scared. I remember crawling into my stepmother's lap, a 30-something mother of two being comforted by a 60-year-old woman. I remember not wanting to leave that safe space.

Back in Hamburg, my first stop was at my Ob-Gyn, where I left feeling increasingly frustrated. I was given an empathic nod but no referrals or resources. I felt that my worries were dismissed. I had the advantage of my mental health training, and I could recognize what I was struggling with. But I felt that I was not taken seriously because too much time had passed since birth, so my doctor did not think it was postpartum depression and anxiety.

I decided to seek out therapy, and as cliché as it may sound, my therapist decided to focus on the relationship with my mother as a possible reason why I was feeling so anxious and depressed. I was starting to feel hopeless and defeated when I reached out to a psychiatrist who specialized in postpartum depression. She referred me to a colleague in the hospital, a psychiatrist who listened to my story and took detailed notes of my symptoms. I cannot highlight how meaningful it was to have someone listen to my symptoms, assess and treat me. And from there, help me take steps toward recovery.

It took me 4–6 more weeks after finding help to start feeling less anxious and depressed; to stop waking up riddled with worry and crying for no apparent reason after dropping my kids off in daycare. It took another 6 months for me to feel like my old self again. I knew I was on track, when I could look myself at the mirror and smile authentically again.

2019

I don't spend much time reminiscing about how life was before parenthood, and how my life was affected by infertility—the physical and emotional scars that it left. Most of them are invisible to the naked eye, like the lingering anxiety I still have on some days, when my chest feels too tight and it's hard to catch my breath. One of the scars I carry is the loss of my marriage. Although this loss was not a direct consequence of our struggle with infertility, my marriage suffered under the weight of this journey.

My life now is filled with listening to my two young boys talk about Superman, Batman, and Legos. They love playing policemen and ghosts. Being mom to two multicultural and multilingual young boys is quite an adventure. I am thankful that I am able to be present for them because I had the knowledge to recognize what I was experiencing, and found a medical team who heard me.

My six-year-old just "graduated" from pre-school yesterday and I reflected about how incredibly marvelous it is be able to experience his childhood with no fear or dread or worry, and no pervasive sadness. I am grateful to have been able to overcome postpartum depression and anxiety, and incredibly blessed to have eventually found the help that was needed.

Into the Darkness

Cormac O'Donovan

I used to wonder what it would be like for a doctor to get fired. It would have to be something egregious, I thought, some catastrophic medical error. I certainly didn't imagine I would be the doctor packing up my things.

I wondered what others thought of me—if they felt pity or some strange sense of fortune. After all, at least it wasn't *them* being asked to leave. I suppose it was easier, in a way, for me to speculate on their reactions rather than turning inward to my own—the guilt and shame of my exile was just too great.

My supervisor had delivered the news after summoning me for a meeting two days prior. There was no agenda, just a sinking feeling as I entered the office. I had tried to reassure myself that I was only tired and emotionally drained; the meeting was probably nothing to be concerned about. After all, you can't fire a doctor for being exhausted, can you?

Administrative leave.

The words hung in the air.

It was a weird confluence of feelings. Failure, to be sure. Appreciation, in some respects, for being spared an outright termination. A bit of relief. How many times had I heard colleagues beg the universe for a reprieve from the daily stress of practicing medicine? Anger, fear, disgust, and sadness—came to help failure make me feel bad. Enjoyment peaked its head out to remind me that I was being disconnected from all the stressors and burned like a small candle to give me a glimmer of hope while trying to grab more of my attention.

I couldn't shake this new image of me: a discarded doctor. It wasn't a sadness that I felt; no, it was despair. How could this happen to *me*? How could I reach a point in my life where my professional identity would become so intrinsically bound to my personal worth? Lose the former and you crush the latter.

And there I was: crushed. Or more accurately: numb.

You'd think in a world of social media, instant gratification, and shelves teeming with books on happiness, that I would've had some message to distract me and shock me out of my despair. *Anything* to get me back on the right track.

> In an office chair, staring at walls adorned with accolades. Awards earned through selflessness and sleepless nights. Funny how my exhaustion had been so glorified until it wasn't.

Instead, I sat in the office I had occupied for two decades, reflecting on my new identity. In an office chair, staring at walls adorned with accolades. Awards earned through selflessness and sleepless nights. Funny how my exhaustion had been so glorified until it wasn't. My boss passed me the document after some trite small talk assuring me my duties would be taken care of. *Who are these people aiding in my kill,* I wondered?

They were going through the motions. *Ha. The motions. What does that even mean?* Colleagues stopped by to offer vapid apologies—like attending the wake of person they met one time—a holiday party or some company picnic. The judgment on their faces was palpable.

As a species, our survival is predicated on our biological wiring—instincts as natural and enduring as the human race. In times of distress, we're born to fight or flee or to tend and befriend. And yet, my less primal side resisted all these options. What was there to fight for? My professional identity had been taken. And to tend and befriend colleagues felt like a fool's errand with disastrous consequence.

A voice enters my head, telling me I deserve my day in court. But I know I cannot be both honest about the reasons for my leave and still be there—respected—for my family and friends who depend on me to be "the strong one."

Another voice comes, "It's not your fault." It's saying the same thing so many others echo—a word of kindness and good intent. And yet it doesn't address the core of the problem, only attempts to dismiss it.

I'm in a defining moment. I can sit in my own self-defeat and wonder who to blame, or take ownership of my story and write a different ending.

In time, I choose the latter—to embrace the self-care I'd been pushing off for years. Now is the time to heal myself so I can one day go back to healing others. It's the most important thing—the *only* thing—I should do now.

Among *The Four Agreements* outlined by Don Miguel Ruiz, he says to be impeccable with your word and always do your best. I need that counsel now more than ever. In this modern age, with all its feigned connection, we remain chronically disconnected, brought together more often by hatred than kindness. We're bombarded with the voices of imperfection and self-defeat.

I know those voices well.

Writers say that the first chapter is the hardest to write. Five years after I sat wondering how life would ever be the same, I'm still writing my first chapter. It's not easy, but it is, indeed, the most important thing I've ever done—the most important story I'll ever write because it's my story. And for those of you sitting in your academic office—with rambling thoughts and unshakeable despair—you, too, can make the next chapter your first.

I didn't think it was possible for me.

Sometimes, it's good to be wrong.

Taking a Knee

Larry Mauksch

My adolescent invincibility dissolved during my junior year of high school. Toward the end of a broadly arched turn, a root emerging through the snow abruptly stopped my uphill ski. The toboggan evacuation after my fall initiated 50 years of patient-hood. The many interactions with healthcare staff combined with my changing relationship with my body influenced my clinical style, teaching, research interests, and family life.

The swelling around my right knee was followed by a series of fluid drainages and eventually the removal of my medial meniscus—all of it. I was in the hospital for a week because the surgeon used an open procedure before laparoscopic approaches were available. After the surgery he asked me to lift my left leg. No problem. Then he proudly asked me to lift my right leg. It would not obey. He laughed and told me how the brain shuts off some muscles when nearby body parts are injured. I felt more like a specimen than a patient with little personal power and in that moment, the butt of a joke. The surgeon did not tell me that I no longer had any cushion between my femur and tibia on the inside of my knee, nor did he warn me about the risks of high impact exercise. For the next 30 years I actively skied, jogged, and played tennis and squash. During the last 5 or 6 years of my racquet sport days my knees swelled after each outing. I regularly iced and used a progression of NSAIDs. For years I viewed pain as an inconvenience, not an obstacle.

In 1997, in the middle of a squash game, my knee suddenly stopped supporting me. By this time, many friends and physician colleagues regularly remarked about how painful it was to watch me walk. My inner bone surfaces had worn away and my knee began to bow out like the leg of a cowboy.

My second surgery came a few days after my knee gave out. My leg emerged with a greater bow as if my horse's girth had expanded. I learned that my bones would continue to wear away. An "un-loader" brace would be needed to straighten my leg, shifting the weight to the outside. The entire preparation for the surgery never included discussion of risks, the increased leg bow, or the need for a brace.

In retrospect, I feel misled and inadequately educated by my surgeons. However, my current appreciation of shared decision making—describing risks and benefits as they related to quality of my life—was not a communication element that I could clearly describe at the time even though I was supposed to teach doctors these communication skills. I was too young in my career, too passive as a patient, and resigned to my condition.

Over the years the pain worsened with increasing bouts of uncontrolled weakness. Involvement in all sports, save swimming and bicycling, stopped. Walking our dog around the block became a challenge. The impact of my severely arthritic knee on family life was increasingly palpable. Our family loves the outdoors—hiking, climbing, and skiing. I gradually withdrew from all these activities. I could not participate in my son's boy scout outings and still feel the loss of what I wanted to share with him. We went on ski trips where my wife and two children would ski all day and come back to our condo to tell me how much they missed me. My knee decay was especially hard on my wife who loves to hike. She never stopped asking me to join her and when I declined she always responded with a combination of empathy and deep disappointment. I felt a combination of guilt, loss, and some resentment that she did not understand what it was like for me. It was obvious that my knees were failing but we all believed that there must be some way for me to overcome this disability.

In my mid-50s the prospect of a total knee replacement became attractive. I read that they lasted 10–20 years and decided to visit a reputable surgeon to discuss planning. The receptionist gave me several pages of paperwork to fill out that I gave to the medical assistant. The resident came in before the attending physician, performed a thorough exam, and was beginning to ask about my reasons for the visit (he never acknowledged the paperwork) when the surgeon barged in. Without acknowledging the resident or noting my paperwork that included my reason for the visit, he launched into a 10-min description of the newest knee replacement technique called "minimally invasive."

"So your knee is pretty bad off. We have a great solution. Our new replacement method (handing me a brochure) decreases time for recovery. Your quadriceps will not be cut."

The term "minimally invasive" struck me as odd as they remove the bottom of my femur and the top of my tibia. When he finished his explanation, still not having asked why I was there, I asked my most important question. "Have there been any changes to knee replacements lasting longer than 20 years?" After a brief silence he said, "No." I had not absorbed his explanations of the new surgery because I was preoccupied with my main question—how long would the replacement last? I wanted to delay surgery as long as possible so to avoid a second replacement.

By this time in my career I understood what went wrong with this visit and it became a story to tell. No communication between medical assistant and physicians. No interest in my reason for the visit. No curiosity about what defined my quality of life. But in the midst of the interaction, despite my understanding of patient centeredness I was a log swept down a stream of one-sided interaction.

At age 59, after postponing as long as possible, I received my first knee replacement. On the first day in the hospital I had a bad reaction to the pain medicine—severe nausea, full body itching. The "pain consult" consisted of a pain specialist interviewing me for 2 min while being silently observed by several trainees who were not introduced. They were lined up at the foot of my bed staring at me. I felt like a specimen again—59-year-old male with pain, itching, and nausea on Dilaudid. No connection existed between all of the visitors and me. I finally interrupted the doctor and said, "Hi, I am Larry, what are your names?" This question broke a rule. The medical students had to speak and the pain specialist was temporality silenced. I felt a sense of satisfaction in gaining momentary control at a time when I felt out of control and vulnerable.

> They were lined up at the foot of my bed staring at me. I felt like a specimen again.

Despite no history of injury, over the next four years I noticed increasing pain in my other (left) knee. Once again, my mobility decreased to the point that I declined invitations to walk or hike. I began using a new brace, received quarterly steroid injections and frequently used NSAIDs. X-rays revealed that most of my meniscal and articular cartilage was gone. This time the same surgeon was much more curious about my experience and my values.

"What is important in your life?" "What do you understand about the risks of this surgery" "What are you prevented from doing that you want to do?"

He even acknowledged how important communication was with patients. Perhaps he knew of my work. Or, perhaps he received feedback about his interactive style. Our shared decision making was more meaningful. I felt cared for and involved in my own care. In 2014, my left knee was replaced.

My experience with osteoarthritis and patient-hood has highlighted many issues that I confront as a teacher, clinician, and researcher. What prevents physicians from being genuinely curious about patient experience and treatment preferences? A powerful combination of forces inhibits young and experienced physicians from sharing decision making, from being curious about patient values, or even expressing empathy. How does time management anxiety affect physician performance? It is crippling and distracts them from being person-focused. Who are the role models in medicine and what is it about them that makes a difference? We know about the "hidden curriculum" where role models openly discount patient suffering and disrespect patient decision-making rights. I devoted the last 20 years of my career to addressing these and other challenges, often reflecting on my patient experience and telling some of these stories to bring scientific findings to life.

I confronted many questions as a clinician. How could I empathize with my patients with chronic suffering while helping them live productive lives? Should I share my own history? How do disabled patients and their family members work together to adjust, compensate, and move forward in life? My curiosity about patient experience, fueled in part by my own experience, helped me acknowledge and accept suffering.

Patients like me cope in many ways. We deny. We use distraction. We rationalize. We use our experience to help others. I was immersed in a naturalistic learning laboratory. My pain, disability, and the dissatisfying experiences with the healthcare system helped me succeed in my professional life.

Now at age 67, I am willing to interrupt physicians to make sure they understand my needs and my questions. As a teacher, I remind trainees that sharing control with patients may be one of their most valuable attributes. We cannot take (patient) suffering away but we can give it meaning and respect. We might contain suffering by helping patients find ways to feel control in their lives beginning with how we treat them in healthcare interactions.

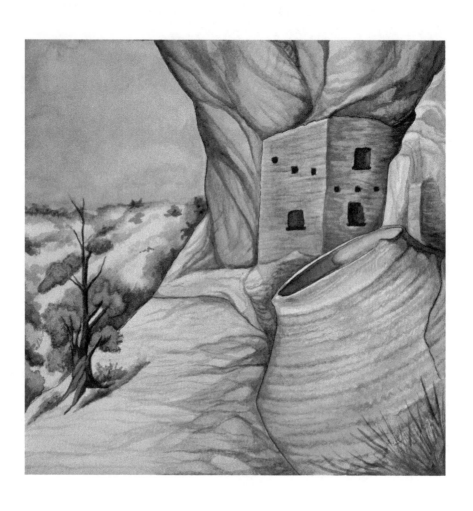

Reflection on Clinician as Patient: Becoming Whole

Juli Larsen

In shopping for some granite, I once saw a sign next to the large slabs that read:

"With any natural stone material, there will be variations in color and markings in each piece of tile or slab. These variations cannot be regarded as defects. They are characteristics of natural stone that give the material its uniqueness and dramatic beauty."

It is telling that variations in stone "cannot be regarded as defects," but variations in people can, and often are, considered defects. In our society, people, who are infinitely more complex than stone, and who have infinitely more variations, are held to a standard of perfection that often curtails the unique and dramatic beauty that could otherwise be endorsed.

As health care providers, we often feel the need to embrace this idea of perfectionism because our patients or co-workers often require that of us. We often want to be seen without defect so that we appear to be legitimate in the eyes of others. Of course, trying to maintain this image only serves to distance us from those we are trying to interact with. In this stance, we are effectively claiming that we are above the human experience. To be ill is human. To be injured is human. To be broken is human. To be flawless is not part of the human experience.

In the pre-industrial revolution, artisans would carefully work to create unique, one of a kind pieces: shirts, belts, plates, blankets. The process of creation gave space for unique characteristics. It was to be expected that no two chairs, bowls, or hammers were going to be the same. These differences were not regarded as flaws, but rather, a feature of that unique handcrafted piece. "Perfect," in this sense, entailed wholeness: a finished, purposeful product.

Enter the Industrial Revolution, where machines were able to mass produce the same shirt, belt, plate, or blanket over and over again, without variance. The concept of perfect changed from wholeness to, without flaw. By using a machine, people could create a flawless item, and "flawless" became our cultural definition of perfect. As a society, we embraced the miracle of flawless, and turned our backs on the substantiality of wholeness.

Would our interactions with our patients, and co-workers look different if we offered wholeness instead of perfection? Would our interactions with ourselves look different if we filtered our life through the lens of wholeness instead of perfection?

Imagine for a moment, being at a craft fair and holding a piece of handmade pottery in your hands. Feel the contrasting rough and smooth textures. See the small grains in the clay. See the way the glaze has covered the piece, sometimes uneven, but creating movement, and light. Sense the weight and substance of the piece of pottery. See, in your mind's eye, the artist's effort and purpose as they shaped and finished that unique piece of pottery. The process of creation allows space for a unique and personalized product. It would seem shallow to view this piece of pottery as flawed or less than because of its original nature. It is this originality—this wholeness, this humble substance—that creates the value, the dramatic beauty, that encourages people to connect with and invest in this product. Perfection isn't even in the equation.

We are the artists of our lives. We can approach life with the lens of perfection or the lens of wholeness. Perfection harbors a critical energy, devoid of safety and risk taking. Wholeness cultivates a humble, compassionate, honest energy. We are able to look at our limitations, whether physical, mental, or emotional, not as faults, but as inherent attributes of being human. Where growth is an option, wholeness invites examination and challenges self-development. Where growth isn't an option, wholeness embraces acceptance, empathy, and compassion.

When we fully step toward the human experience, we are free to acknowledge and openly examine what we lack - the "holes" that we possess. Wholeness allows us to take those wounds, those "holes," and with humility, patience, and com-passion, and reach toward our potential.

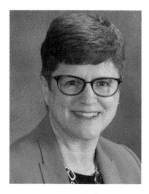

Colleen T. Fogarty MD, MSc, FAAFP, is the William Rocktaschel Professor and Chair of the Department of Family Medicine at the University of Rochester Department of Family Medicine. She earned her MD degree at the University of Connecticut School of Medicine in 1992. Dr. Fogarty is considered an expert in writing 55-word stories and using them as an educational tool for self-reflection. She has published many of these stories, poetry, and narrative essays in several journals.

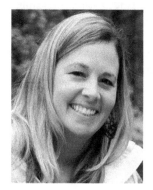

Aimee Burke Valeras PhD, LICSW, is faculty with the NH Dartmouth Family Medicine Residency. She completed her Doctorate in Social Work from Arizona State University. Dr. Burke Valeras recently coedited the book Integrated Behavioral Health in Primary Care: Evaluating the Evidence, Identifying the Essentials. She lives in Concord, NH with her husband and three children and enjoys riding her e-bike and hiking.

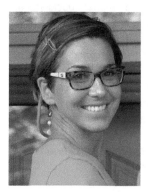

Kathryn Warren Hart DDS, is a pediatric dentist at Marillac Health in Grand Junction, CO. She completed a residency in pediatric dentistry at The Children's Hospital, Denver, CO in 2008 and an AEGD Residency at the VA Hospital in San Antonio, TX in 2004. She has taught dentistry students at CU and at Pacific Schools of Dentistry. She enjoys audiobooks, family and friends, and of course, flossing.

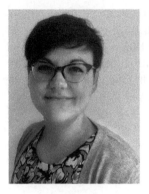

Rachel L. Hughes PhD, LMFT, is the Program Manager of Sea Mar Everett Child and Family Services. She completed her doctorate in Medical Family Therapy at Saint Louis University. When not at work Rachel loves to read, travel, bike, and explore her home city, Seattle.

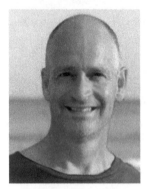

Tai J. Mendenhall PhD, LMFT, is a Medical Family Therapist and Associate Professor in the Couple and Family Therapy Program at the University of Minnesota (UMN) in the Department of Family Social Science. He earned his doctorate from the UMN in 2003. Outside of work he enjoys motorcycling, home-remodeling, and traveling with his wife, family, and friends.

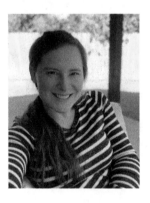

Grace Pratt PhD, LMFT, is a digital packrat, an aspiring plant lady, and the mom of Henry (born in 2015) and identical triplets Alex, James, and Luke (born in 2017). She has been the Behavioral Medicine Faculty at Integris Great Plains Family Medicine Residency in Oklahoma City, OK since she earned her PhD in Medical Family Therapy from East Carolina University in 2014. Her research and clinical interests center on couples, trauma, infertility, and high risk pregnancies, as well as the neurobiology of healthcare provider burnout and resilience.

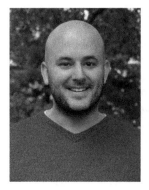

Jonathan B. Wilson earned a BA in Psychology from Oklahoma Baptist University, a MS in Human Development and Family Science from Oklahoma State University, and a Doctorate of Philosophy in Medical Family Therapy from East Carolina University. He spent 6 years teaching graduate courses in Marriage and Family Therapy, and has provided individual and relationship counseling in various outpatient mental health practices, as well as inpatient behavioral health. He's a published author (journal articles and several book chapters) on various topics including attachment, intimacy in relationships, and family therapy, and he has ongoing research interests in the area of intimate partner violence, family systems, attachment theory, and integrating medical and behavioral healthcare. Jonathan has also presented his research at multiple state and national conferences.

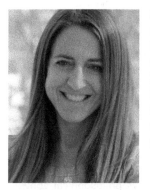

Samantha Pelican Monson PsyD, is a psychologist and primary care behavioral health consultant with Denver Health in Denver, Colorado. She completed a doctorate in psychology at University of Denver in 2009 and has a certificate in primary care behavioral health from the University of Massachusetts Medical School. Outside of work she enjoys international travel, hiking out her back door, both water and snow skiing, and relishing time with her husband and twins.

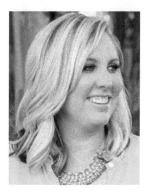

Jamie E. Banker PhD, LMFT, is an Associate Professor at California Lutheran University. Dr. Banker completed her PhD in Human Development and Marriage and Family Therapy at Virginia Tech in 2010. Her primary clinical and research interests are women's and family health. She has published research on community trauma, young adult sexuality, best practices for training systemic therapists and psychotherapy interventions. Outside of work she enjoys spending time at the beach with her husband and sons.

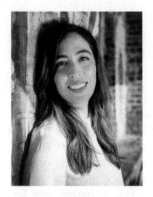

Tania Riosvelasco MA, MFT, works in private practice in Hamburg, Germany. She completed a master's in Marriage and Family Therapy at the University of San Diego, CA in 2010 and is currently working towards becoming a certified Emotionally Focused Therapist. She is a proud mom of two multicultural kids and enjoys yoga, awesome food, and naps.

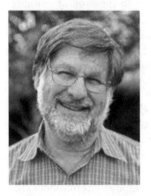

Larry Mauksch M.Ed, is clinical professor emeritus at the University of Washington Department of Family Medicine. He completed a masters degree in school and counseling psychology at the University of Washington. Over 30 years he worked as a clinician, teacher, researcher and author in primary care and behavioral health. In retirement he enjoys time with family and friends, travel, woodworking, reading, hiking, biking, cross country skiing.

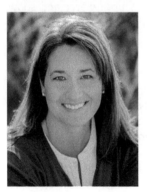

Juli Larsen BS, C-MI, is a meditation instructor in Grand Junction, CO. She completed her undergraduate work at Brigham Young University, majoring in Health Promotions. She enjoys philosophical conversations with her husband, discussing good books with her 5 children, and spending precious quiet time swimming and gardening.

Death and Loss

Electronic supplementary material The online version of this chapter (https://doi.org/10.1007/978-3-030-46274-1_6) contains supplementary material, which is available to authorized users.

Death and Love.

Endings

Colleen T. Fogarty

Disheveled hair; gaunt frame
Writhing–
Moaning–
Suffering
Pain–

Pleading...

Tears

Family vigil
They come from close and away
Hushed voices
Reminiscing
Pleading...
***
Life snuffed out
Unjustly too soon

Crash...Drunk driver
Stray bullet...Bystander

Alone in a new land....
En route to work...
Heading to college...

Estranged and unknown
Or, remembered lovingly

Loss
The void remains

Professional Growth Through Personal Suffering

Sabrina Mitchell

We exit the elevator at floor 6, the familiar antiseptic smells of a hospital filling my nose. My mom guides me down the hallway to the room where my brother and sister are waiting. I'm 22 years old, in the midst of completing medical school applications and I've just arrived on a flight from San Diego, with a return ticket already booked for the next day. As we walk down the hall, thoughts in the back of my mind from "how will I afford another plane ticket for the funeral?" to "what if he lives through this…again?" We arrive at my father's room. At first glance, it seems like this is different from the times I've done this before, but I am not yet convinced.

In the hospital bed lies my 49-year-old father, an ex-green beret medic, his hospital gown unceremoniously and somewhat embarrassingly tangled about his waist. Ankles and wrists tied to the four corners of the bed, Foley catheter pulling taut as he tries to wrestle and wiggle his way, to where I do not know. His oxygen mask has slid up his face and now covers his nose and most of his eyes. As I move closer to him, I see he has bitten through the plastic on the lower portion of the mask.

When I lean forward to talk to him and try to fix the mask, he snaps his teeth as if to bite me. He looks at me, eyes wild yet pleading, and shakes his head no. I look at my mom who shares that he wouldn't keep the nasal cannula in so they put a mask on him. This is the second mask through which he has chewed.

Over the next few hours it becomes increasingly clear that this time *is* different. This is the last time we will ever do this.

The years of my dad's ailing health are coming to an end. Finally? That word sits quietly in the back of my mind, but I do not share it. My dad has suffered from ill health since I was eight years old. But the last 4 years, while I've been in college, have been the worst. Hospitalized several times a year, most frequently at a Veteran's Administration hospital that is 400 miles from my hometown, where my parents live, but somewhat conveniently located on the campus of the college that I am attending. Now here we are again, sitting around his bed, but for a visibly different reason. This time my mom will not be taking him home.

The doctors seem relieved that my mom agreed to make Dad a DNR, so that when his heart stops they won't do anything to try and bring him back. This relief was surprising to me as we knew and accepted that he was dying. It was then that I learned sometimes families want to try anyway no matter how grim the outlook.

> The years of my dad's ailing health are coming to an end. Finally?

My dad continues struggling in the bed, pulling and moaning. In an effort to comfort him, I pull my chair as close to the bed as I can and lower the side rail carefully, which gives him enough movement with his arm to get the oxygen mask off of his face. I lay my head next to his, my arm across his chest, and he quiets.

"Help," he whispers to me.

"What do you need?" I ask him, but he can only repeat, "Help."

The nurse comes in to check on him and gives me an angry look. She informs me that I can't put the bed rails down and that Dad needs to leave his oxygen mask on. I explain to her that the mask doesn't seem comfortable for him and that I can't reach him with the bed rails up.

"Do you want him to fall?" she asks

"I'm not sure how he can fall. He seems very weak and you have him tied to the bed," I respond without returning her sarcasm.

She walks around the bed, between my dad and me, raises the rail, then leaves the room. My dad becomes more agitated so I slide my arms between the bars, to hold him again, which quiets him for a time.

As the day progresses Dad becomes increasingly confused and agitated. Intermittently he moans, struggling against his restraints, unable to find comfort. The moaning becomes louder. When the nurse comes to check on him again, I ask if he can have something, anything, to help him be more comfortable.

"He's already had all he can have," the nurse replies, no apology in her voice, no compassion in her eyes. I plead with her to ask the doctor what more can be done.

"If we give him anymore, he'll stop breathing and die," she says to quiet me.

"In case you didn't notice, he IS dying," I retort, my voice rising with anger and grief. "That's why we are all sitting around his bedside." The nurse shakes her head and leaves. Later she returns with my father's next shot, given in his butt instead of his IV, to try and make it last longer.

By now the moans are nearly continuous. It is too much, even for our veteran crew of bedside sitters. We have started taking shifts, one or two at the bedside and the others in the family waiting room at the end of the hospital ward. The respite in the family room is minimal, as my father's cries can be heard throughout the ward. I do not know for whom I feel worse: my father, who is clearly suffering and incoherent, or all the other patients and their families who have to listen to this man cry out for hours without the background of love and respect that we, as his family, bring to this dismal situation.

Finally, 8 pm comes; visiting hours are over and we are told that we will have to leave. It was both horrifying and relieving to hear, but we didn't seem to be bringing him much solace with our presence anymore.

My father did not die that night. The next day, the tug of life came. My brother, sister, and I had to be back at work or school the following day.

Two days later, the call finally came. The call we had fought against for many years and then prayed would come a few days before it actually did. I do not know if my father died suffering, as I witnessed. I suspect so, but my mom has spared us those details.

Even 23 years later, my emotions surrounding this event are powerful...sometimes even raw. I still remember the sense of relief I felt when mom called to tell me that it was, at last, over. This is the death my father suffered. This is the type of death I fight to spare my patients and their families. This is the death that shaped my approach to patients and families before I had even started my first year of medical school.

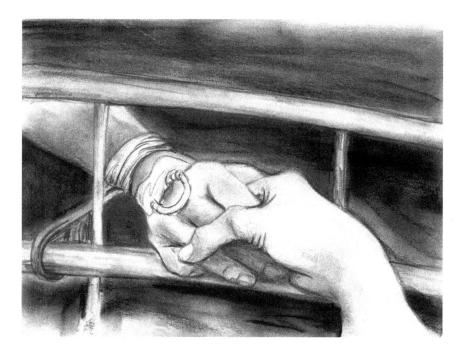

Walking with Grief

Keith Scott Dickerson

Walking in the high desert open space behind my neighborhood was the most soothing and sustaining activity I could muster in the days that became weeks after my Mom's unexpected death. The steady, almost automatic cadence and crunch of each footfall, puppy at my side, was the only time I felt at ease, both tuning out my distress but also promoting deep pondering on this turn of events.

Weeks earlier I had taken a quick mountain bike ride on this portion of trail when I had taken "The Call"—the one we all dread as our parents age—from my sister. I had dropped to my knees that evening upon hearing "Keith...our mom just died," and at that spot, the next day, I built a small rock cairn memorial, inconspicuous, that I am sure most folks walking these trails don't even notice. In the initial weeks after her death I deliberately plotted a route past this memorial many days, stopping each time to say a prayer for strength to endure, and express thanks for our relationship. While walking, a variation of the song from the movie Finding Dory would play in my head—"Just keep walking, just keep walking." It was a metaphor, and my reality, at that moment.

My mother lived her life as fully as possible, doing what she loved, until her last breath. Among her many activities she regularly volunteered as a pianist at the age of 89. The story of her last moment, and last song, is remarkable. On a Wednesday evening at her retirement community, she finished dinner with her boyfriend and walked to the chapel to play piano for an evening service. Her boyfriend stayed at her apartment, watching the service on closed circuit TV. As he watched from her living room, my mom finished the opening hymn—The Old Rugged Cross—and she lurched forward, then keeled over backward, landing on the floor, a gasp rippling through the congregation. The pastor heard all this, rushed up to the piano, and had the presence of mind to remember she was DNR/ DNI. A quick assessment revealed she was dead and the pastor honored her wishes to allow a natural death. This was the first lesson I would discern as I stumbled along my grief journey, namely, the importance of making your end of life wishes explicit and widely known.

In the weeks following her funeral, I found myself telling many of my patients her story. Many folks I take care of in clinic, and on our inpatient teaching service, are in their 80s and 90s. Before her death I had used examples from my mom's health travails to build rapport, make connection, and bring home key points about health with my older patients. I've shared aspects of my life's joys over the years and telling my long-time patients about her death only seemed fitting. Each patient that I shared with had the same reaction—it is what they would ideally want for themselves, namely dying while still active and vibrant. I am thankful to have included my patients on my walk with grief.

Even though I agree that it was the proverbial "good death," the unexpectedness and not being able to say goodbye was and is challenging. I am quite mindful that many folks in the world and even within my own family have endured and suffered much worse circumstances and loss. It was a blessing that I had long-standing adult relationships with both my parents; still the sudden loss, and loss of the second parent, was an existential crisis for me.

As I had for my father, I delivered the eulogy at the memorial service. It was a learning experience both times—finding out details about their lives, gaining perspective on their core being, reconciling mixed emotions and long-standing hurts. All the while I worried about striking the proper authentic and loving tone, and wondered about holding it together while baring my emotions so nakedly. Bitter in the pain of the mournful passing of an irreplaceable relationship, sweet in the remembrance and honored gravity of the situation. I also acutely realized that, as by far the youngest child in my family, I may well live through each of my siblings' deaths. This has motivated me to do my part to sustain and deepen my relationships with them.

While sharing my Mom's death with patients felt right and I believe did deepen the therapeutic relationship, there has been a shadow side. When I now take care of an older patient, especially one who is my Mom's age or older, I have to admit I have an acute pang of anger and resentment at...what? The universe? Fate? God? Why is this person still alive, but not her? What did she and I miss out on by not being able to work through a less sudden demise? There was no cathartic, tearful good-bye, no holding of hands, no life-encompassing embrace. It is a stark reminder to live each day as if it could be our last–that whatever can happen at anytime can happen today. Grief is hard, necessary work.

Over time it was hard not to notice that some folks walked along with my grief more helpfully than others. What I mostly found was that after the initial out-pouring of cards and sentiments, precious few checked in with me. There were a few notable exceptions, which deepened our relationship in a way that they will probably never realize…until they experience grief. I came to recognize that we as a society, and as individuals, are very uncomfortable dealing with grief in an ongoing fashion as opposed to the acute aftermath. No one knows what to say. You are afraid to stir the pot—what if the person breaks down?

More than anything I realized a deficit in myself. I had not reached out to folks over the years. I resolved to do better going forward, and have adopted a tradition of my Mom's. After her death I found out that she had forwarded a classic quote from Dietrich Bonhoeffer to others who were experiencing acute grief. I made up some cards with this quote and try to remember to share it with friends and family who have suffered recent loss, and offer it here in the same spirit:

There is nothing that can replace the absence of someone dear to us, and one should not even attempt to do so. One must simply hold out and endure it. At first that sounds very hard, but at the same time it is also a great comfort. For to the extent the emptiness truly remains unfilled one remains connected to the other person through it. It is wrong to say that God fills the emptiness. God in no way fills it but much more leaves it precisely unfilled and thus helps us preserve – even in pain—the authentic relationship. Furthermore, the more beautiful and full the remembrances, the more difficult the separation. But gratitude transforms the torment of memory into silent joy. One bears what was lovely in the past not as a thorn but as a precious gift deep within, a hidden treasure of which one can always be certain.

Sundays have been the hardest. I moved away from home when I was 18, reveled in the independence, and did not keep in touch with my parents all that well in my 20s. I grew to understand, value and sustain a vibrant relationship with them. After my father's death I very much further solidified my relationship with my mom, settling into a routine of a weekly Sunday phone call, often lasting an effortless hour. I often find the void of loss opening up on Sundays, then realize… it's Sunday. She was my biggest supporter, always interested in what I was doing. While going through her belongings I found a folder with every letter I had sent her, along with newspaper clippings of my accomplishments. Of course I miss not having our weekly conversation, and that is OK.

My mom's death has been an existential jolt to my sense of place in the universe, while the subsequent bereavement has been a self-journey toward understanding what I value, and why. As the Bonhoeffer quote correctly notes, it is not realistic to expect the void to be filled. There is a sting of pain, but also a sweetness in the memories of a lived love. More than ever I believe that bereavement is a normal process that must be lived through, confronted, or coddled as needed. It is not something to be numbed nor medicated. Disciplined attention to self-care such as daily walking or running, eating well, playing music, writing stories, engaging in relationship, and doing pleasurable activities have been major grief modulators.

Last week I realized a month or so had passed since I had plotted my dawn walk past the memorial cairn in the desert. I felt the pull to traverse that path. Shockingly, I was 50 yards past the cairn before I realized I had walked by it, absorbed in my quotidian thoughts. I doubled back, a moment of panic, wondering if it had been destroyed, whether it was still there—how had I missed it? There it was, intact, no need for repair. I had walked my way past grief.

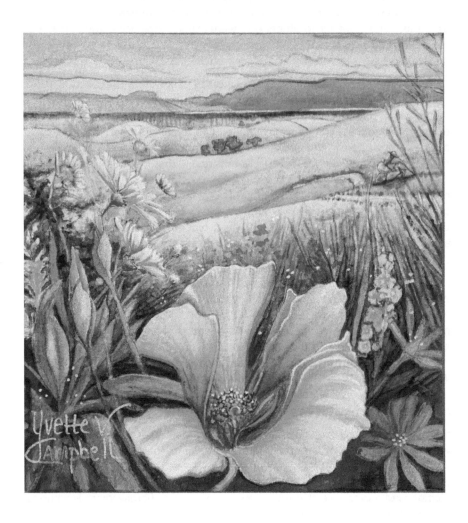

The White Rock in the Desert

Sally Stratford

A roadrunner drowned in the pool that morning.
I was too young to understand
why we couldn't swim with it,
    that long tail of brown feathers.
Mom took me for a walk instead, to look at rocks in the wash.

We crawled through a hole in the fence
behind the condos, climbed down
into the dry river bed among smooth ovals and loaves.
The desert was purple in early April.
Shrubs and rocks spread up the slope of Smoke Tree.
When we stopped to notice rabbit pellets and gourds,
I asked if we could really drink water from a cactus.
The rocks in the riverbed were black with silver specks,
and gray like heavy bird eggs.

We picked them over, hefted them through.
And quite naturally, my mom explained
that he had been very small.
About the size of my favorite doll, Sara,
who slept in the top drawer of my dresser.
She said he only breathed for two days, but with help.
She and my dad held him, all wrapped up,
for his final few minutes.

I spotted the reflection of a white rock.
She picked it up and turned it over in her hand.
It was clear and shined in the sun.
She said we would keep it and put it on his casket
along with moss and daffodils.
She didn't say, but I knew the rock glowed
because it had been touched by Jesus, for us.

Years later, I sit on my parents bedroom floor with a manila folder, pictures
of a baby taped with tubes,
a hospital band small as a hair tie,
and a paper with his hands and feet
stamped in purple ink, each one with six fingers and six toes.
My thoughts go to that desert walk, so far away,
and the rock still glowing
so far beneath the cemetery grass.

Daughter or Doctor? The Exquisitely Unique Pain of Watching a Parent Die

Deborah Edberg

The death of my mother was sudden and unexpected. She had been in good health for a 74-year-old woman and we had a delightfully innocuous conversation that morning while she was on her daily walk.

"It was an undiagnosed cerebral aneurysm that ruptured," the Emergency Room attending told me over the phone. I had 8 hours in the car to review all the potential scenarios. She was alive but disabled, she was fine, she was dead. I arrived at the hospital at 3 am. The Neuro ICU resident on call showed me her CT scan. "Here is where the aneurysm was. You can see the clips here and here. There you can see a slight shift." There was no way to miss an entire side that was obscured in white.

"Can I see her?" I finally asked. "Yes, yes, of course." He showed me to her room.

Her hair was perfectly colored yet slightly out of place from the blood crusting on her left temple. The tube in her mouth distorted her lips and her eyes and face still wore the remnants of her perfectly made-up look from earlier in the day. "Never leave the house without a full face," was what she had always told us. "You never know who will see you if you're in an accident, God forbid."

"Hi Mom. I'm here now. You had a little bit of a stroke and you're in the hospital now. We're going to take care of you..." My voice broke as I held her hand and she seemed to squeeze it a tiny bit. We sat together for a while until I left and went to our family home to rest.

As I lay in my childhood bed that night next to my husband, I thought about the years spent growing up in that room, always with my parents sleeping on the other side of the wall. Mom had been fiercely proud of my going to medical school. She bragged about my career shamelessly, inevitably inflating whatever minor successes I enjoyed. It felt like such a betrayal of her faith in me that I hadn't known this would happen. Had her lifelong migraines been a symptom of something more? What about the pain in her legs over the past few years? I felt like I was slowly slipping into an abyss. It was impossible to imagine life without my mother.

Over the next week, she seemed to gradually improve. She was increasingly aware of my and my sister's presence, opening her eyes and squeezing our hands in answer to specific questions. We put pictures of her and her family around her bed hoping if we gave the nurses a personal frame of reference they would feel more attached to her and give her a little extra care.

> Having missed the signs of her aneurysm followed by the signs of her secondary strokes and recognizing the endless real or perceived opportunities when I could have impacted this course, I felt ultimately shamed and hopeless.

At the end of the week, they tried to extubate her, but her throat had swollen so much around the tube that she ended up gasping for air and they had to sedate her to reintubate. When she became less responsive after the reintubation, we thought she had been over sedated. A new team took over to cover the weekend and we asked them several times if they thought her level of sedation seemed excessive. We didn't want to push too hard in fear of alienating them from us and from her care.

On Monday, however, when the original team came back on, they recognized that this was a significant change from her baseline and immediately ordered the MRI that showed the secondary strokes she had suffered as a result of vascular spasm that is common after a significant bleed like my mom's. It signified a much graver prognosis and a more difficult recovery if she were to live.

For the next week, we tried a few different options, but in the end, the neurosurgeon called a family meeting. My sister and I shared full Power Of Attorney to make decisions on her behalf. From prior conversations, we were very confident of her wishes and agreed to withdraw care.

The guilt I felt over this course of events was devastating. The memories of her boasting of my skills as a physician hung over me like a grotesque shadow. Having missed the signs of her aneurysm followed by the signs of her secondary strokes and recognizing the endless real or perceived opportunities when I could have impacted this course, I felt ultimately shamed and hopeless.

I was determined to make up for it by carefully orchestrating the scenario for the end of her life. Having navigated the care of many patients in the withdrawal of care, I felt confident this was where I could be a successful and informed advocate for my mom. I asked to talk with the hospice service to ensure that she would be comfortable at the end. The hospital administrator assured me the ICU nurses were well trained in withdrawal and the hospice team wouldn't be necessary. They had a protocol to follow. Conflicted, I again fell into the role of wanting to be cooperative.

When we arrived at the hospital they had moved mom to a more private room in the ICU in the corner. They had a morphine drip set up and a lovely young nurse with a sympathetic smile. I asked if the doctor would be present and she assured me it wouldn't be necessary. My sister said a tearful goodbye and left my husband and me together in the room.

And so we began. The nurse explained the protocol—she told us she would inject a small amount of morphine before removing the NG tube and the ventilator tube. I asked her about the swelling in mom's throat and if it would be uncomfortable for her to have the tube removed. She reassured me she would be comfortable. And then she removed the NG tube.

For the first time in a week, Mom's eyes shot open, she looked at me with what seemed to be pure panic. I grabbed her hand and looked at the nurse desperately. "This is a normal reflex," she told me, but she didn't seem sure. "Is the doctor here?" I asked but again was told no, the doctor wasn't generally present for extubation. Then she took out the ventilator tube and Mom began to gasp for air. "Can you give her more morphine?" "Well the protocol only allows for us to increase it every 5 minutes" she told us and walked out of the room. I held onto Mom's hand and looked into her panicked eyes. "I'm here," I told her and rubbed her hand. "Please..." I called out to the nurse, "can't you give her more morphine?" The alarms at the bedside began to go off as Mom's heart rate went up and her oxygen level decreased. The nurse came in to silence the alarms, but they sounded again several minutes later. "Can't we turn those off?" I begged her. "The protocol...." she told me. I saw her on the phone and then she came in and increased the rate of the drip. "Let me give her a little bit more..." she said. I pleaded with her. "She's dying, can't we just give her enough to make her comfortable? You can see she's gasping for air..." Mom's hoarse gasps were amplified by her swollen larynx, her entire body was wracked with the desperation.

We finally pressured the nurse to give her higher doses of morphine. When Mom's body ultimately relaxed and her pupils constricted I kissed her and said goodbye. My husband and I sat in the waiting room before going to see my sister. The horror of it all was stunning. The entire event had lasted about 20 minutes, but it had been an eternity. My sister didn't ask us what had happened and we didn't speak of it again.

That afternoon we planted lilies for her in her garden and when my father asked if her death had been peaceful, I stared out the window as I told him "yes". I packed up my room and some old family photos. We shared stories about mom with neighbors and friends. I tried to get out of that room in the ICU but every time I closed my eyes I saw her panicked face. My identity as daughter and doctor, forever entwined, were decimated.

Returning to work was a challenge. I had been off for three short weeks for the entire experience and was back in the office a week after her death. Initially, rounding in the ICU with the teaching service was nearly unbearable. Over time, I was able to tune out the alarms and focus on my service. I leaned on my colleagues to gain perspective when patients presented with headaches and stroke symptoms so I wouldn't continue searching for the aneurysm I had missed in my mother. When my father died 10 years later I pushed hard for hospice care and was able to support him in having the peaceful death at home he had wanted.

As a physician, I thought I would have the knowledge, skills, and resources to advocate for excellent health care for my parents. But for my mother, I am eternally haunted by my shortcomings in her care.

When I think of my mother now, it's more often the way she laughed at our jokes, the way she worried about our choices, and the way she gave her wise but often unsolicited advice. It's less now that I see the panic in her face during those final moments, but I don't think that memory will ever totally be gone.

As a physician, my confidence was rocked harder through this experience than with any patient under my own care. As much as we try to distance ourselves from our role as physicians when we are in the role of a loved one, it is nearly impossible to forego one for the other. And whether we become deeply entwined or coldly distanced, it seems unlikely we can ever reach the exact right amount of space. For me, I will think of my mom's pride as a goal for which I will strive in my journey as a physician. I may not always represent the doctor she thought that I was, but I can try to get pretty close.

A Cosmic Perspective on Death

Paul D. Simmons

I carry a coin in my pocket every day. On one side, there is a quotation from the Roman emperor Marcus Aurelius which he wrote to himself in his personal diary: "You could leave life right now." On the other side, an hourglass, an iris bulb, and a skull remind me of the passage of time, the shortness of life, and the inevitability of death. The words "Momento Mori" surround the skull —"Remember You Will Die."

The nitrogen in our DNA, the calcium in our teeth, the iron in our blood, the carbon in our apple pies were made in the interiors of collapsing stars. We are made of starstuff.

Carl Sagan

I am made of calcium, iron, carbon and other atoms, every one of which were formed in the intense gravitational pressure at the core of stars that explosively died billions of years ago, billions of miles away. When I die, my atoms will return to the world. Other animals, plants, and rocks will use them, then die themselves. I am made of borrowed materials. At some point, the loan will come due, and I'll have to give it all back. Does it seem odd that I find constant reminders of my death and Sagan's cosmic view comforting? As Michel de Montaigne said, "To philosophize is to learn how to die." My own explorations have led me to draw comfort, not from the popular refuge of faith, but from the perspective of science and secular philosophy.

By the sweat of your face you will eat bread, till you return to the ground, because from it you were taken; for you are dust, and to dust you shall return.

Genesis 3:19

How can we face the inescapable truth that everyone we love and know will die and be returned to dust? Not only do I have to give back my borrowed materials, my loved ones do, too. Every relationship you and I have is temporary, yet we hardly live like it. Marcus Aurelius and his fellow Stoics remind me to imagine, every time I embrace someone I love, that they are already dead. "When you embrace your child, you are embracing a mortal," they say. That sounds harsh, doesn't it? But there is deep comfort in a reminder to be grateful for every moment—to be thankful that I had these beloved mortals in my life at all, and to "give them back" with gratitude (despite the tears) when the time comes.

I do not fear death. I had been dead for billions and billions of years before I was born, and had not suffered the slightest inconvenience from it.

Mark Twain

I have no reason to expect that my consciousness will survive my own death. I have no reason to believe that the people or even the pets I have loved are somehow "out there," waiting to meet me again. Still, I am grateful and amazed that I got to know and love them, given the remarkably long odds against any of us existing. I should play my part on the world's stage for as long as I am given, and when the hourglass runs down, I hope to be comfortable—not only physically but existentially—leaving the stage when the time comes. Others are waiting in the wings to play their part. That's all easy for me to say, but the ultimate test of any philosophy is how it holds up when in the crucible of pain, suffering and death. "To philosophize is to learn how to die."

Death does not concern us, because as long as we exist, death is not here. And once it does come, we no longer exist.

Epicurus

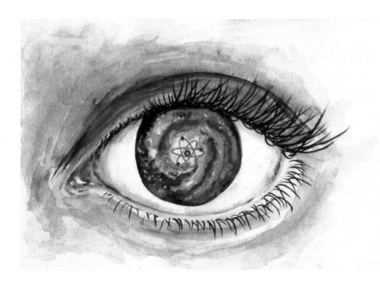

Rather than collapsing like a dying star into my own singular grief when I experience a loss, I have been comforted by a cosmic perspective, which provides me with a sense of wonder at my own small beginning and eventual ending; my own tiny contribution to the cycle. I'm humbled by and grateful for the gift of consciousness for this brief moment, and the gift of loving others even transiently. I am hopeful that this understanding can comfort me when my own ending comes —that it is also part of the Whole, the next necessary step, the giving back of what has been briefly borrowed. Momento mori.

Can We Call This a Death?

Stephen W.B. Mitchell

My son Bo died on October 8, 2010, he was 14 weeks old. Typically, it is after this statement that I feel a rush of shame, embarrassment, and uncertainty. I can hear the recipients of this data calculating in their minds, tapping out the numbers on their mental adding machines, 14 weeks? Wait a minute; he was not a real kid. In our medical and cultural nomenclature, Bo was a tissue that underwent a fetal demise or spontaneous abortion.

Now, before I make some people anxious or angry let me clarify. This is not a political narrative and I am disinterested in starting a debate about when life begins in the womb. Rather this is a narrative about loss and how we come to define what our losses mean. You see, when my wife Erin and I miscarried Bo our loss felt like a death. Yet, we have felt, in so many different ways within the medical and societal contexts around us that we cannot call this loss a death. Thus, the meaning we have come to regarding our medical event of miscarriage has been denied. In so many ways, it feels that we have to wrestle with these two larger contexts of medicine and society to be allowed to grieve. And so, Erin and I find we are constantly asking the question can we call this a death?

You might be familiar with this scenario. Erin and I went back and forth about whether or not we were "ready" to have a child. At various times in our first 3 years of marriage, we alternated between the position of being the partner "ready" and "not ready." Back and forth the discussion went. We finally arrived at the same decisional destination when I had said I was "ready" and Erin had a month where she felt pregnant but found out she was not. Her level of disappointment about not being pregnant surprised her and indicated to her that we were both in fact "ready."

Quite naively, in retrospect, we gleefully set about getting pregnant and "starting a family." Things went as planned. The first month or two of trying resulted in a positive pregnancy test and we moved from "trying" to "we are having a baby!" In some respects, everything felt easy and under our control. We started planning financially for a child, buying clothes for a child, making a place in our home for a child. Erin paid attention to her health, tried to sleep, tried to eat *the right thing*, and we got books to educate us about being parents. We were planning for the life that was, that would be, and we were ensuring that it would all go smoothly.

I think that since Bo's death we have wondered about the societal narrative that "if you do all the right things and have a great attitude you will have a perfectly healthy baby." Things went smoothly until violent morning sickness. Erin experienced a daily ritual of waking up before 5 am to get ready for her hour and a half commute to work. She would rise, feel nauseous, dry heave into the toilet, take a shower, dry heave into the toilet, drink ice water (water without ice made her feel nauseous), dry heave into the toilet one more time and head off to work. At work, she felt constantly exhausted and when she came home at the end of the day she would come into the house and immediately fall asleep on the couch for the rest of the night. This was our daily routine for three months and it did not feel good to either of us. Erin frequently would express consternation about no one telling her being pregnant could feel awful and I felt like I had lost my wife. We no longer hung out and talked at night or were able to enjoy any of the outdoor activities we liked. Erin simply was too tired and sick to function as we both expected.

Pregnancy altered our lives in so many unexpected ways that felt negative and hard. This was not part of the "if you do all the right things and have a great attitude you will have a perfectly healthy baby," narrative. In our lived experience, every corner of our existence was being influenced by pregnancy and our lives were already changing as if Bo had been born. At times we wondered, "Are we already parents because we feel like we are doing parent like things." Things like sacrificing our own interest, feeling like our marital relationship had to grow with a new person now in the mix, and the emotional and psychological energy we were committing to integrating this new entity, person, into our daily lives.

Our imaginations were running wild about our new life and our hearts were filling up with life. We wondered who Bo would be, what he would look like if he would be a good skier but also we began to measure life 4 weeks, 5 weeks, 6 weeks, and so on. When we went to our midwife she felt Erin's belly, took measurements, asked about diet and weight gain all to assess how life was developing. This felt like life, like newness, a fresh start, blood and tissue, physical, emotional, spiritual, the creation of someone beautiful, a living moving reality. Bo was this deeply beautiful amalgamation of hope and wonder mixed with discomfort and struggle. In so many ways this is what life is, the combination of good things and bad things, positive and negative colliding.

Then, life died. The Doppler touched Erin's belly and our ears were met with the horrifying static of white noise. The familiar sound of a galloping horse that is a heartbeat in utero was absent. Where was Bo? Our lives went strangely numb, tingling with fear and the refrain, "This can't be happening to us," continuously echoed in our hearts. Then it moved between us, spoken, as we drove dumbfounded to the hospital for a confirmatory ultrasound. Our midwife told us, "You will either find out everything is OK or you will find out you miscarried." We feared the reality that would be ours but hoped with the smallest speck of possibility that all would be OK.

There are no words to describe the feeling of these *in between* moments from Doppler to ultrasound. Agony and despair. I saw them on Erin's face and felt them in her spirit. Her body, the vessel that she had been trying to understand and adjust to for the last 3 months had introduced another twist. Where had control and *doing the right thing* gone now? She was silent and slowly sinking into darkness. I saw it, I felt my own despair over what might happen and a deep fear about whether or not Erin would be OK.

But everything was not OK. Melissa, the ultrasound tech, met us in the hospital waiting room and took us back to the exam room. There life was, it popped up on the screen so suddenly without any fanfare, or at least there life was supposed to be. But it wasn't. No movement, no heartbeat. I remember at that moment my heart and body was overwhelmed with love. I didn't expect it, I didn't know it would happen but instantly I heard my heart whisper, "I love you." I loved that life that was no more. Erin and I sat in that dimly lit exam room and wept. We wept like you do when someone you love dies. Can we call this a death?

We exited the hospital and entered a new *in between*. The *in between* that comes when death visits and grieving begins. This is an "in between" with no foreseeable end. This liminal place is where a decision about what to do with the body must be made. But in a miscarriage the question is how do you want to get the body out of your body and then dispose of it? This is one of the unimaginable things about miscarriage. There are no societal narratives and no medical formulas for the dissonance that wells up with this decision.

Erin felt something mysterious happen when she got pregnant. As a disembodied observer, all I can do is try and communicate what I saw and what she said to me about being pregnant. Erin described both a physiological and psychological presence that began to grow inside of her the moment she saw the double lines materialize on the pregnancy test. Her body instantly felt different and she became aware that she was now sustaining something, someone, in her body. The cruel reality of miscarriage is it contradicts the physiological and psychological change that was growing within Erin. This life she was to sustain for 10 months needed to be released from her body at 3 months 2 weeks. It either needed to be released through birth or extracted through dilation and curettage. Both felt antithetical to Erin's senses and in some ways felt like a deep violation of her body and the role of mother that was developing in her psyche. Thus, the decision of what to do with the body felt complicated and incongruent.

We chose to give birth at the hospital, but it's not giving birth to life, it's giving birth to death. Nothing made sense or felt as it ought. We could say we chose to pass the body but you pass kidney stones not a life that has ended. The doctor told us we were passing fetal tissue but Bo felt like more than fetal tissue. Tissue does not alter your entire existence as ours was being altered. The nurses took us as we came and allowed us to say Bo was more. In fact, one nurse gently shared that she too had miscarried and expressed her own confusion about what had happened. She acknowledged that after all the years since her miscarriage she still felt "in between" the death and grief. The right words to describe such an abrupt ending continually returned to death. It all just felt like death. An abrupt gut-punch and the sudden cutting off of joy and hope.

Misoprostol assisted with inducing labor and after waiting through a long ago-nizing night Bo moved through Erin's body as the morning sun rose on October 9. We gently cradled his 4 inch and 0.07 ounce frame in our hands and our hearts cracked like shattered glass. The nurse that was with us at the time looked at his genitals and said, "Well, that looks pretty penial to me." We couldn't disagree and our son was named Bo. Staring at his developing frame I marveled at his fingers and toes and eyes. His little rib cage and body rested on my skin and I couldn't help but think, "You just came too soon buddy." Life had once been there but now death resided. I looked at Bo and said, "Bo we know you are not here but we need to say good-bye," and so we sang over him, prayed over him, blessed him, wept over him, kissed his head, and let go of him to never hold again. Our first greeting was a farewell.

The farewell lingers. It lingered in Erin's body as she bled for 4 months following the miscarriage. Her milk came in, and in her bodily confusion about the birth that was really a death, she developed a painful case of mastitis. It lingered in our hearts as sadness and depression crept in and confused our daily lives.

Even now as I reflect on what happened nine years ago I feel the grief. When Erin and I miscarried again in 2016, it was impossible not to remember Bo and those same feelings of shock and sadness. I look at my three boys and watch them play together and there is this presence I cannot shake, this sense that at any moment their other brothers will come tearing out of the house into the fray and play along. I look at my three boys and am reminded that people ask all the time, "How many kids do you have?" I never know what to say. Three, five pregnancies, three kids what are my options? How do I let you know that there is more here than meets the eye?

Can we call this a death?

Unimaginable Loss

Julia L. Mayer

The sharp ring of the heavy old telephone startled me. Everyone in the waiting area seemed to freeze. On the third ring, I got up from my blue plastic chair and crossed the orange carpeting and cautiously lifted the receiver. The impatient voice on the line asked for me. I had been waiting, suspended in time, for an update. I could barely speak. I recognized the voice of the female surgical fellow on the other end of the line.

She told me, while I stood in front of strangers in that dingy waiting area of the state-of-the-art Manhattan heart hospital, that my mother was not going to recover. Hemorrhagic pancreatitis she'd unexpectedly developed after cardiac bypass and aortic valve replacement surgery was untreatable. The fellow told me that I was allowed to see her, which meant I could enter a curtained area where her body lay hooked up to machinery whose sole purpose was to keep her alive—or at least keep her body warm—until the rest of my family could arrive to say their goodbyes.

My siblings, father, aunt, and uncle and I gathered around her bed. We took turns trying to find something to say that might represent at least a little of how each of us felt. In our shock, the words did not come easily. Mostly, we stood silently. After the intensive care staff disconnected her, I held her hand until it grew cold.

It was 2008, shortly before my 44th birthday. I had an inkling that I'd be greatly affected by my mother's death, but I didn't realize for a long time the tremendous impact it would have. During the first few months after her death, I couldn't stop seeing intrusive images of the orange-carpeted waiting area or my mother's bloated body covered in tubes and tape. I'd jump whenever a phone rang. People made fun of me for what seemed to them like an excessive reaction to a common noise. My heart racing, I'd be swept over by a terrible wave of dread. I knew what the symptoms were and why they were happening; I just couldn't stop them.

I'd been a clinical psychologist in practice for nearly 20 years at the time and could recognize PTSD in myself. I did what I could to process the traumatic events by telling my husband and close friends the details, purposely walking through them in my mind repetitively, and grounding myself in the present. But I couldn't help being exhausted, anxious, detached, and forgetful. I recognize those features of my state only now in retrospect. At the time, I just felt overwhelmed without words for it.

> I sifted through my feelings and beliefs and gave myself the time to experience the complex, contradictory array of emotion that is grief. I slowly began to return to my life.

I thought I could handle returning to my private psychotherapy practice quite soon after my mother's death. The first patient—an anxious, kindly woman in her 50s whom I'd treated for several years—asked me how my time away was. I answered that it was "nice." I heard myself say the word as though from far away. I knew that she was terrified of losing her own mother who had been ill and I couldn't bring myself to say that I'd just lost mine. I was afraid I'd cry uncontrollably in our session, that the balance in our relationship would shift. I felt that it wasn't ethical to inject my external life into her treatment. I was in way over my head. But I believed at the time that I was okay.

Before I was to see this same woman the following week, I found myself dreading our appointment, wishing she'd cancel, longing to be safely home in bed. I struggled to hear her as she spoke about her mother's illness. I was bored, distracted, impatient, and irritable. I hid it as well as I could. I'm certain I was not doing my best therapy. I was either stuck in my head, which was full of horrors and memories or trying to control the impulse to cry.

But other psychotherapy sessions felt like an escape from my pain. I looked forward to those. A young, recently married woman I'd seen for a year for anxiety began to have flashbacks of early sexual abuse with her father. She needed additional weekly sessions to manage her overwhelming feelings and process her traumatic memories. By focusing on her trauma, I was able to keep mine at bay. Our efforts to put her memories together like puzzle pieces from the past were compelling and rewarding. She was emotional, and, at times, I was as well; her story was so frightening and sad. I felt rage at her father for harming her as a child. I tried not to express it except to validate her feelings. I had a glimmer of awareness that some of my rage didn't belong to her father but instead had to do with my own grief.

Ultimately, she began to understand what happened to her and its impact. There was grief in her work about her father not having loved her in a healthy way and of the loss of her happy childhood. This was a different kind of grief than mine and I was eager to do the work with her, believing we were making good progress. But after our appointments, I'd immediately find myself plunged into my own misery again. I'd rationalize that it was good for me to use my work as a psychotherapist to escape in this way. It took months for me to realize that I was not allowing myself the time to grieve fully.

Around this time, several of my friends became impatient with me. They seemed to feel that after a few months, an adult should be done grieving her mother's sudden death. Of course, they had not yet lost their own mothers. They knew that my mother and I hadn't always had the greatest relationship. One repeatedly suggested that I go back into my own therapy. She found it annoying that I wasn't much fun and she didn't want to hear about my struggle anymore. One friend vanished from my life, probably unsure of how to support me or whether she wanted to. I was unsure of how to negotiate these relationships. I did reluctantly meet with a therapist.

I learned that I had powerful guilt feelings. I believed that somehow I should have saved my mother. I'd often been a caregiver to her in the past. My attachment to her was always an anxious one. I loved her intensely, but I also hated her. She'd been cruel to me at times, couldn't tolerate vulnerability in me, and was highly judgmental. I had retriggered feelings of anxiety going back to a much older trauma of a baby brother who died of sudden infant death syndrome. I sifted through my feelings and beliefs and gave myself the time to experience the complex, contradictory array of emotion that is grief. I slowly began to return to my life.

As the months passed, I continued to make time for my grief. I cried with family members. I visited the grave. I looked at pictures, told stories to people who wanted to hear them and gradually began to accept that my mother was actually gone forever and that my relationship with her would always be there anyway and would always be complicated.

My ability to be present with my patients improved. I could be sensitive to their experiences of loss. It became evident to me that many kinds of losses can lead to a need for grieving. Current losses can tap into feelings of old grief from past losses. I found that I now had it within myself to help my patients make the space for their own complex and sometimes unacceptable feelings of grief. When a patient experiences a major loss, I can now tell them that there is no time frame —that the sadness lasts forever, only it becomes softer. I can help them grow from their experience as I had.

Today, 10 years after her death, I can still imagine myself back in that hospital waiting area. I can hear the frightening noises, feel the panic, and see my mother in the curtained room with tubes taped to her beat-up body, her essence gone. Losing my mother had felt unimaginable. Over time, I've gradually accepted it along with my own complicated and contradictory feelings about my loss. Now, as I join my patients in their journeys through loss and grief, I understand their experiences more deeply than I ever could before my own loss. I know better how to give them the guidance, compassion, and reassurance that they will come out on the other side, older and wiser.

What Do You Need Right Now?

Karlynn Sievers

I saw there wasn't a heartbeat before she did. One of the drawbacks of being a pregnant physician, I guess.

My obstetrician knew that I was nervous about this pregnancy. I'd had three miscarriages before this one, all early, and even though we were past the point where my other pregnancies had failed, I was still nervous. I think that's what prompted the ultrasound—"just to make sure everything is OK," she said. And in a few minutes, there was my baby on the monitor. Arms, legs, head, spine—all perfectly developed. She went to taking measurements and calculating growth, engrossed in her task. I think that's why I noticed it first. The four chambers of the heart, but no fluttering movement among them.

"Look," she said. "I always think they look kind of like a gummy bear right about now, with their arms and legs so small. And here's…oh."

My heart skipped a beat with the unspoken confirmation of what I'd already seen.

She referred me right away for a formal ultrasound. "Sometimes I miss things. Maybe I had a bad angle with the ultrasound. I want to confirm that I'm right before we take any action." But I knew the drill. How many times had I sent women for formal ultrasound myself, "just to get confirmation" that the thing I already knew was true? Hoping that I really did just have a bad angle with the ultrasound probe, or that I just didn't get the right view of the baby.

They were able to work me in for a formal ultrasound 20 minutes later. I drank as much water as I could before the appointment to make sure my bladder was full. Maybe it just hadn't been full enough, that last little vestige of hope said. Maybe it was something as silly as being dehydrated from a busy morning clinic—a funny story I'd tell someday about how I didn't drink enough water and scared myself and my doctor. No need to call my husband yet. The ultrasound tech chided me anyway. "You were supposed to drink a lot before your appointment—your bladder isn't full at all." And in the end, it didn't matter. She wouldn't tell me there wasn't a heartbeat, because "I'm not allowed to say anything until the radiologist reads the films." But I could read the ultrasound for myself.

"I think I want to just wait and let things happen naturally," I said when my OB/GYN called me with the news. I had done this before, and I knew what was coming. And there was something that felt noble about going through the process of miscarriage. It was like a tribute to the life that my body wasn't able to sustain. "You've never been through something like this," she assured me. "Your other miscarriages were early. This one will be different." We bargained for a while, but she talked me into a D&C. After all, I needed to work. I was on call all weekend, and I had patients scheduled in my clinic that next week who needed me. And how would I tell my co-workers that I was pregnant, but I'm not now, and I need some time off? We would schedule the procedure on my post-call day, and no one would be the wiser.

That call weekend was busy, which felt like a good thing at the time. No chance to dwell on the fact that I still felt pregnant—still had nausea, the fatigue, the feeling of fullness in my stomach. Not much time to register the lullaby that played overhead each time a baby was born in the hospital. No real chance to be jealous of the obviously pregnant women that suddenly seemed to be all around me. Not much time to worry about the procedure itself (would it hurt? How would I feel before and after? How was it possible that I had counseled women about this so many times, and didn't feel like I knew what to expect myself?) I had to step out of rounds at one point so I could pre-register for my upcoming procedure. A woman with a very kind but hurried voice ran through her checklist of questions, designed to speed up my check-in on the day of the surgery. What procedure would I be having? Do I have any medication allergies? What is the state of my health?

"Is there any chance you're pregnant?" she asked.

"I don't know how to answer that question," I responded.

"Oh...."

And then it was the day of the procedure. I went to sleep pregnant and woke up not pregnant. Just like that, it was over. They put me in recovery on the pediatric floor so I would be less likely discovered by my colleagues—to avoid explaining to everyone why I was in the hospital. The nurses came and went from time to time, but I didn't need much, so they mostly left me alone. My husband stayed home with our son because we didn't have a sitter. My room looked out over the park, and since it was Christmas time, I mostly watched the Christmas lights from my window, shining from the snow-capped trees. I knew from working on the labor and delivery floor that the OB rooms looked out over the same park. I wondered if my baby would have enjoyed them.

Fortunately, my surgery was uncomplicated, so I recovered quickly and was able to go home that afternoon. The next day I saw a full clinic of patients, placed orders, wrote notes as if it were a typical day. My obstetrician and I agreed that I didn't need a scheduled follow-up appointment—I knew what to look for, how to tell if things were going wrong.

And just like that, I was back to my "normal" life again. Quietly, I recovered (both physically and mentally) from the miscarriage. Almost no one knew that it had happened, and the ones who knew didn't know what to say to me. It made it easy for me to conceal it, to keep it silent and personal.

My story turns out to be a happy one. I eventually went on to have a wonderful, healthy son who completes my family in a way I could never have imagined. And I'm not bitter or resentful about the experience at all. Quite the contrary—I feel grateful that people worked so hard to protect my privacy in a situation where it could have been easily compromised. But I sometimes wonder if things would have been different if I hadn't been a physician. Would I have been more likely to tell people what was happening? Would there have been more support for me if I had? Would they have forced me to take time off to recover? Would I have wanted it if it were offered?

I don't know the answers to any of these questions. But I do know that I try to get my patients to answer these same questions for me in the middle of their own losses and misfortunes. "What do you need right now? How can I support you?" I hope it makes me a better doctor, and that it is a fitting tribute to the life of the baby I never got to meet.

Caring for Our Loved Ones

Randall Reitz

I never cry.

That's not true. I only cry when dogs die.

Some of my most poignant memories are of watching my dad choke-up reading *Old Yeller* and *Where the Red Fern Grows* over breakfast and experiencing the same tears when I shared these classic dog stories with my own children.

——

Norris and Venna Miller met during high school and married 1 week before he entered active military duty. This Utahan landed near Utah Beach and spent several years in France, including time as a prisoner of war. They had two children before he joined the Korean War. After his return, they had a third child, a miscarriage, and a girl who only lived 1 day. They adopted 2 babies who were brought to them through small-town arrangements with their family doctor.

Bob and Helen Reitz met in Utah shortly after he finished a degree in civil engineering at the University of Nebraska. They couldn't afford a house, so they built a garage. Their family of 7 inhabited these cramped quarters as they hand-crafted their house in the evenings over the next two decades.

These 4 people, my grandparents, have all died now.

Bob died first. Despite his clean-shaven jaw and crew-cut head, he was all Santa Claus in his whiteness, roundness, and jolliness. I loved to bounce on his lap as he taught me to fish and whittle. The scent of his hot chocolate, sausage, and sourdough pancakes coaxed me awake whenever I slept over. His death was unexpected, of a stroke in 1997. He'd been replacing shingles on the roof earlier that week.

Helen died next. She was a feminist before her time. She was one of the first female graduates from Brigham Young University and had a career in special education. Having survived the Great Depression, she was miserly with her resources but generous with her creations. The family ethic could be described as "Fix it up, wear it out, make it do, or do without." She was always professorial in her cat-eye glasses, 60s clothes, slender frame, and wise observations.

> I pray that I'll benefit from the same compassion that Moab experienced.

She lived to be 85 and spent the last year in a nursing home. By then, her warm intelligence had rotted to paranoid dementia. She frequently accused us of abandoning her. The daily log of visitors and conversation topics that we diligently recorded in her room failed to persuade her otherwise. My mom believes she eventually died from self-starvation.

Norris died third. His grandkids loved him because of his caring bluster. He would always greet us by introducing his fists: "Meet Iron Mike and Dynamite Dan. If you're not on your best behavior they'll knock you into the middle of next week."

He eventually succumbed to age. His family kept him at home for as long as possible, but his last years were stripped through cognitive and physical decline. My last memory of him is of a brief visit to his VA nursing home. When I greeted him in a shared living space he had clearly lost 50 pounds and was tucking his head and his self under the collar of his shirt. In the delirium, he didn't recognize or acknowledge me or my mother, his daughter. We left with him still wild-eyed and hiding in plain sight.

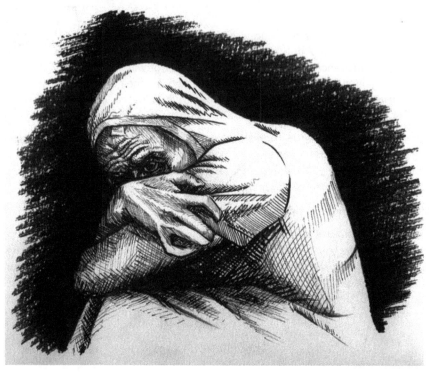

Venna died last year, at 93. She was a dedicated housewife and church leader. With her flinty pioneer spirit, she ran an orchard, garden, and chicken farm, canned her own food, milled her own soap, baked famous pies, and ran a bustling sewing business out of her home. She mowed her own lawn until 92, the same lawn that had hosted my parents' wedding nearly 50 years earlier.

She lived at home until her death, but depression and dementia robbed her house of joy. When she made it out to attend a family event, she would often fib that she'd baked the store-bought pies and would start asking to be driven home shortly after arriving. By the end, we could never leave her alone and we had to disable her car and stove after life-threatening incidents. Despite constant care, she had two gruesome falls in her last week and died with large bruises marring her beloved face.

While the sudden news of Bob's stroke was definitely the most dramatic, the tortured decline of the others was far more traumatic. I've concluded that only Bob had clearly had the good death that the others were denied. Don't get me wrong, there really was no other way. Their values and religion removed any option other than suffering slide until their bodies and minds reached terminal collapse.

—

Now, despite my years being half the final ages of my grandparents, I can already sense the creep of memory loss. It is my genetic birthright. I recognize that my brain is constantly searching for words it once summoned with ease. In earlier years, I never took notes in meetings. But now, without them, I'll forget decisions and assignments. I hope that I'll keep it together to see my children marry and create grandchildren for us to enjoy. But, I feel it coming, and am preparing.

—

My family has a beloved dog, Moab. Sixteen years ago, a family friend found her at the town dump and asked us to adopt her. The first week her ribs were a washboard, her face a muddy scab, and her reflexes all flinches and winces.

Over the years she was our loyal companion on trail runs, family vacations, and in 4 homes. She snuggled with us in bed, barked at visitors on the porch, and filled our lawn with poop.

About 3 years ago, she started slowing down. At first, she would get farther behind on long runs. Her trails ended for good when she followed the wrong group and we needed to search for an hour to find her.

She eventually lost her senses of sight, smell, and sound. We could no longer take her on vacation, but she and our cat did very well at home. This last January, we came home from travels and found her locked in a closet. I don't think she'd been there long, but coming out she was running into walls, lost in a home that she'd known for years. We held a family meeting and concluded that it was time to take the step that we'd avoided for months. I called our veterinarian and scheduled an appointment to end Moab's life.

The night before was dedicated to her. We prepared her favorite food, took pictures together, loved on her, and shared treasured Moab stories. The next morning the children shared their final words with Moab: "You've been the best doggy." "We can never replace you." "I hope you don't suffer anymore."

My wife, Ana, and I drove her to the vet in a quiet, sad minivan.

It was obvious that the office staff understood the nature of the visit because they spoke in reverential tones and ushered us straight to the exam room. Our vet came in, expressed his concern for us, asked a few questions, and described the procedure to assure that we were fully informed. We signed our consent and he stepped out of the room so we could be alone with her.

Five minutes later he returned with two syringes. He again affirmed our commitment and then applied the first injection. This one caused her to sleep within a minute. We lifted her up to the table and he applied the second injection.

He instructed Ana and me to place our hands on her side where we could feel the warmth of her heartbeat and the rise and fall of her breath. Over the next minute, these movements of life slowed until they stopped entirely. Her fur cooled. The vet checked her heart with his stethoscope and confirmed her death.

It felt odd to walk out of the office without her. On the drive home, we both felt calm in the conviction that we'd ended her pain and confusion. Perhaps because of this assurance, I didn't cry that day. I was confident that we'd done right by her.

I pray that I'll benefit from the same compassion that Moab experienced: that my personal physician will be afforded the right to assist in my final medical procedure. I hope that my loved ones will support my decision to stop living before my organs stop working, that they will embrace me with their hands, absorbing the last breath from my lungs and the last beat from my heart.

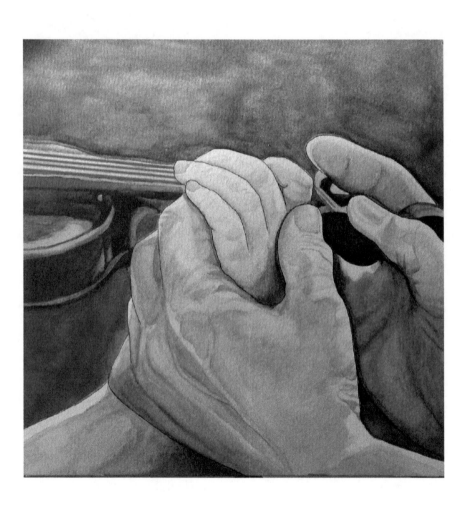

Reflection on Death and Loss: Music of Life

Juli Larsen

We have all sat in the safety of a large concert hall, watching as the house lights dim and the concertmaster tunes the orchestra before the conductor assumes his position of relative anonymity, back toward us, baton in hand. We have watched as that baton, like a marionette puppeteer, guides and coaxes beautiful music from the instruments. We have seen the lights shine off the polished wood of the cello and tracked the miniscule movements of the violin bow as it teeters between the strings. We have watched the upper bodies of the musicians sway, heads bobbing, hair bouncing, eyes fluttering, as they feel their way through the music.

The conductor, now pounding the rhythm of the gallant march and then, transitioning with both body and mind, becoming diminutive in his movements, backs down to the softest of sounds - the singular aching of a violin played, quiet, secure, drawn out, and likewise our breath is pulled out of us, as that note hangs in the air. We close our eyes, letting the vibrations of that last note wash over us. Breathing in the resonance, we express gratitude for the offering.

We often experience life like we experience music. We cheer the crashing brass of a marching band, we reverberate with the drum line at a football game, we fold ourselves into the security of a lullaby, and we pace ourselves like the stalwart beat of an old church hymn. Music is life and life is music.

What happens when the music ends? What happens when the last exhalation is offered?

We struggle. We yearn for more. We listen. We remember. We talk. We share. We question. We mourn and we try to remember once again.

When we try to remember the great music that has touched our lives, what do we remember? Few, if any, of us will actually remember the individual notes, the complexities of the harmonies, the dissonance, or even the faults of the musicians. What we remember about music is what we felt and experienced when we listened to it. The music is catalogued in our mind and heart not as a set of black and white notes that were correctly or incorrectly played; rather, we remember the music as a feeling: peace, excitement, happiness, suspense, and gratitude.

And so it is with the life of a loved one, whether that be a family member, a dear colleague, a childhood pet, or perhaps a patient who has had a deep impact on our life, we remember the feeling of their life. The same could be said regarding the loss we feel when a meaningful experience comes to a close, the loss of a significant relationship, or the loss of an opportunity. We remember the feelings of the experience, relationship, or opportunity. We mourn for the loss, the connection we felt with that person or that experience. In this process of mourning, this raw desperation to somehow regain a piece of what we had, in this reaching, we begin to recognize more clearly the music that surrounds life.

Each life, each experience, each opportunity presents itself to us with unique musical qualities, some come crashing in on us, some provide a steady beat, some seem unresolved and dissonant. As the last notes are played, we reflect on the music of life, no longer trying to hear each note, to see if it fits in, or compliments the rest of the score, but we become more contemplative about the meaning of each note. We listen as each note begins to represent a point of decision, each measure the unfolding of an emotion.

As we learn to listen to the music of life, the people around us, the experiences that surround us, we begin to hear life in a way that the spoken language cannot comprehend. It becomes a form of communication without words. It is a language that is felt, rather than spoken. In that feeling, rests the nobility of life. That nobility is the gift that washes over us, the figurative last note that hangs in the air while we close our eyes and breathe in the resonance of it.

In our human experience we will all come face-to-face with death and loss, in a variety of forms and with a variety of emotional impacts. In those quiet moments of uncertainty and silent struggle, we breathe. We pause and breathe in the music of life that surrounds us, allowing the nobility of life's music to flow through us and around us. This music may no longer be a music we hear, but it is a music we will forever feel. It is beautiful music, this life we live.

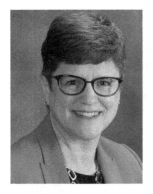

Colleen T. Fogarty MD, MSc, FAAFP, is the William Rocktaschel Professor and Chair of the Department of Family Medicine at the University of Rochester Department of Family Medicine. She earned her MD degree at the University of Connecticut School of Medicine in 1992. Dr. Fogarty is considered an expert in writing 55-word stories and using them as an educational tool for self-reflection. She has published many of these stories, poetry, and narrative essays in several journals.

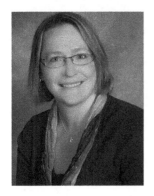

Sabrina Mitchell DO, is the Program Director at the St. Mary's Family Medicine Residency in Grand Junction, Colorado. She completed her doctorate of Osteopathy at University of New England, College of Osteopathic Medicine in 1999 and Family Medicine Residency in 2001 at Sparrow-MSU in Lansing, Michigan. The formative moment shared in this book set the course of her practice in medicine. Outside of medicine she enjoys riding her Harley alongside her husband, spending time with her children and crocheting Star Wars characters.

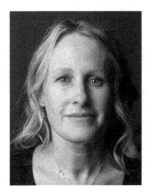

Sally Stratford Deford poems have been published in Dialogue, Tar River Poetry, and Fire in the Pasture: An Anthology of 21st Century Mormon Poets. She received her bachelor of arts in English from Brigham Young University. She enjoys fine art photography, trail running, plays the upright bass in a bluegrass band. She lives in Grand Junction, Colorado.

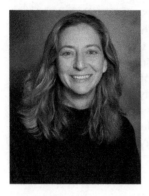

Deborah Edberg MD, is the Director of Graduate Medical Education Development at Rush University in Chicago. Prior to that she was the founding program director of the McGaw Northwestern Family Medicine Residency Program in Humboldt Park. She received her medical degree at Sidney Kimmel Medical School and completed her Residency in Family Medicine at the University of Connecticut. Outside of work she enjoys traveling with her family, scuba diving and rescuing Bernese Mountain Dogs.

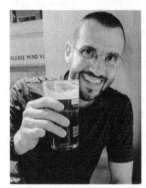

Paul D. Simmons MD, is a faculty physician at the St Mary's Family Medicine Residency. He received his bachelor's degree in History from Baylor University in 1995, and his medical doctorate from the University of Colorado School of Medicine in 1999. After several years of practice in rural settings, he has been teaching residents since 2010. Outside of work, he enjoys CrossFit, trail running, obstacle course racing, Stoic philosophy, and his pets—all of which are impermanent.

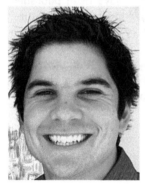

Stephen W.B. Mitchell PhD, LMFT, is in private practice in Atlanta, GA. He completed a doctorate in Medical Family Therapy at Saint Louis University in 2017. Stephen works with his wife Erin to help couples tell their stories of loss as a means of healing and connecting with one another. Outside of work he enjoys being with his family in the outdoors.

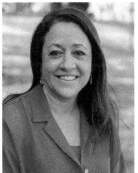

Julia L. Mayer PsyD, is a psychologist in private practice in Media, PA. She received her bachelor's degree from The University of Pennsylvania and her Psy.D. from Widener University. Author of the novel, A Fleeting State of Mind, and co-author of the 2016 book, AARP Meditations for Caregivers, she also has a weekly psychology and social justice podcast, Shrinks on Third.

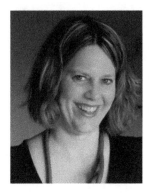

Karlynn Sievers MD, is a faculty member at St. Mary's Family Medicine Residency in Grand Junction, CO. She completed her MD at the University of MO—Columbia in 2001. While she has published articles in Conn's Current Therapy 2020, 5-min. clinical consult, and FP Essentials, this is her first narrative work. Outside of work, she enjoys reading, gardening, and spending time with her husband and two sons.

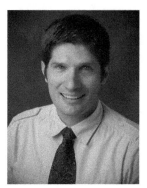

Randall Reitz PhD, LMFT, is the Director of Behavioral Medicine at the St. Mary's Family Medicine Residency in Grand Junction, Colorado. He completed his doctoral studies at Brigham Young University. Outside of work he enjoys trail running with his wife, mountain biking with his children, and baking with his thoughts.

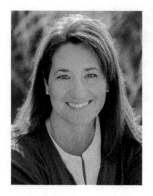

Juli Larsen BS, C-MI, is a meditation instructor in Grand Junction, CO. She completed her undergraduate work at Brigham Young University, majoring in Health Promotions. She enjoys philosophical conversations with her husband, discussing good books with her 5 children, and spending precious quiet time swimming and gardening.

Lightning Source UK Ltd.
Milton Keynes UK
UKHW020828110123
415103UK00002B/19